WILD MEDICINE
Spring

Other books in the series

WILD MEDICINE
Spring

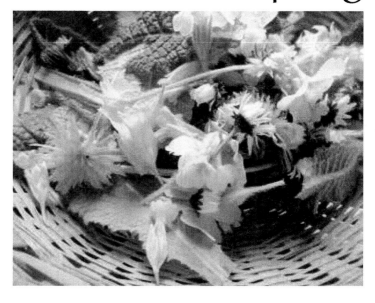

Ali English

Aeon Books

Disclaimer

The intent of this book is solely informational and educational. The information and suggestions in this book are not intended to replace the advice or treatments given by health professionals. The author and publisher have made every effort to present accurate information. However, they shall be neither responsible nor liable for any problem that may arise from information in this book.

First published in 2020 by
Aeon Books Ltd
12 New College Parade
Finchley Road
London NW3 5EP

Copyright © 2020 by Ali English

The right of Ali English to be identified as the author of this work has been asserted in accordance with §§ 77 and 78 of the Copyright Design and Patents Act 1988.

British Library Cataloguing in Publication Data

A C.I.P. for this book is available from the British Library

ISBN: 978–1–91159–769–8

Printed in Great Britain

www.aeonbooks.co.uk

Contents

Spring

vi   Contents

About the Author

Herbalist Ali English has been passionate about herbs from a young age and went on to study herbal medicine at Lincoln University, graduating in 2010 with a BSc (Hons). Since then, she has set up a practice in Lincolnshire that focuses on offering herb walks, workshops and a variety of related services, in which she tries to convey her love of our native herbs and wildflowers to anyone who will listen. *Wild Medicine: Spring* is her third book, with many more to follow.

Acknowledgements

For Matt, my Viking – as always an unconditional pillar of support and love.

And for the plants – those friends and neighbours who bring such delight and who provide pretty much everything we really need in life, as well as giving such beauty to the world.

Preface

Welcome to *Wild Medicine: Spring*. Spring herbs are an absolute delight, coming through as they do after an often long, monotonous winter and bringing with them vibrant greens and yellows; and even though damp, rainy and often chilly weather may often preclude gathering and drying herbs at this time of year, nonetheless a plethora of useful and tasty recipes can be made with what you can pick. It is a particular joy to walk the countryside at the very threshold of spring, falling as it often does during late February in the UK, though late snow can often laugh at us for being deceived. Watching the world slowly stretch awake, one bud and sprout at a time, defying snow and late frosts, is a constant delight, and our native herb life is well equipped to deal with these challenges. Early spring light on the first mornings without frost seems redolent with promise, lying in golden swathes across the land, lifting and heartening the spirit and slowly calling the earth back into life again. Slowly the sun regains its warmth, the birds begin to sing, and the season gathers pace, bringing us meadow flowers, hawthorn and the onset of the greener season.

This book is meant to give you a starting point for learning to know and appreciate the herbs of spring, from the sunny flowers of dandelion – intrepid explorer and denizen of vegetable beds, flower beds and gravel areas – across to the rampant scramblings of cleavers and the juicy leaves and starry flowers of chickweed. Later in the spring there will be cowslips and violets to delight the eye and soothe the body, and later still, on the cusp of summer, there will be hawthorn flowers, all of which make wonderful medicine, alongside many others.

It is my hope that these seasonal books will provide a source of information and kindle a keen delight in the glories of our native plants, both those growing in the hedgerows and those weedy adventurers tucked into nooks and crannies in our own gardens. Plants have long been a passion of mine, ever since a bespectacled girl child of 13 asked for a garden and was given a small, round plot with four herbs and a sundial in it, plus a copy of Culpeper's *Complete Herbal*. Three years on, that small plot boasted more than 40 herbs, and I was badgering my mother for more space. The obsession went on from there, and, many years later, I graduated from university and began building a career working with the plants that had delighted, inspired and enchanted me for so long. It is difficult to ever feel alone in the world if you cultivate a friendship with the local wild plants – everywhere you look, you will see them eking out a living for themselves: the wily and determined dandelion tucking himself into cracks between paving slabs, the tall, elegant willow and balsam poplar by the river in my home city of Lincoln, hawthorn in the hedgerows, poppies in brilliant red swathes across farmland in late summer. Plants are all around us, and over time they have become a true need for me, like water and food, air and freedom. Indeed, they are deeply entwined in my very blood and body, as they are for all of us – we inhale as they exhale, and we exchange breaths with plants constantly, sharing the same air.

It is my aim that these books will provide hedgerow travel companions to inspire and console you through the winter and, perhaps, to tuck into a pocket and take along with you in the warmer seasons. May they give you many years of enjoyment and help you towards your own deepening friendship with the plants that surround us and give us so much.

Green Blessings, and happy foraging!

North Lincolnshire, 2020

Spring

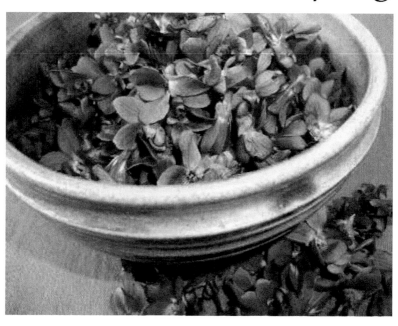

Introduction:
foraging and medicine making

Spring can be an exciting though sometimes frustrating time of year for medicine making, starting off slowly with mists and frosts and soggy days, then suddenly speeding up as the sun gains warmth. Nevertheless, even as early as February, there are quite a few wonderful plants that are well worth making the trek for through rain, chill, early fog and wet ground. Here are a few things to remember if you would like to spend time gathering herbs in the spring for drying, or for medicine making in general.

Foraging

In the dampness of very early spring, the likelihood of being able to find surface-dry herbs is extremely low, so I recommend having a dehydrator handy, if possible, plus a selection of old tea towels to wrap herbs in. A salad spinner can be a handy gadget too if you bring in herbs that are very wet indeed. Hanging surface-wet herbs up to dry is, sadly, pretty much impossible in the spring as they tend to mould instead of drying, so the dehydrator is a handy alternative. Dry your herbs in a single layer, on a low to moderate setting, and keep track of any water trapped in pockets on the leaves – I find that the best bet is to get as much water off as possible on a tea towel before you lay the herbs out in racks, and possibly even use a salad spinner to remove the worst of the water first. Also consider other ways of preserving the early spring herbs: make tinctures and vinegars, freeze them, or incorporate them in soups and stews.

I rarely gather aromatic herbs in the early spring for drying, not least because their scented compounds haven't usually come through enough yet to make it worth while. Wait until at least late April or early May for scented herbs, in order to let the plants get more sun and produce more volatile oils: by this point you should also find that there is a greater likelihood of getting a dry day to pick them.

There are some plants that can be gathered for roots in the spring, most notably wood avens (*Geum urbanum*) – which rather goes against everything we know about root gathering generally. These roots can be gathered in late March, April or early May, ideally in full or partial sun, so that the scented compounds in the roots have more time to gather strength. Wood avens is an annual, so if you wait until autumn, you will find that most of the nutrients in the roots have been used to produce flowers and seeds. Digging them up in early April guarantees the best possible harvest. Just use the same principles as any other root harvest – dig them early in the morning or late afternoon, cut off the green tops and bunch them up for drying, then scrub the roots clean, pat them dry and chop them up. They should dry quite readily on saucers or put into the dehydrator if they aren't too small – and can then be stored for use later in the year, or tinctured.

Flowers are often picked in the spring, often independently of the leaves; wide, shallow wicker baskets or hydroponic hanging drying trays can be useful pieces of equipment if you want to preserve some of the delicate fragrance often found in spring blooms. Gather the flowers on a warm day and spread them out in a single layer in the basket, flicking the basket in the air every other day to turn the flowers over, or brush your fingertips over them to turn them over. Some of the smaller flowers will shrink considerably as they dry: for these, you may want to line the baskets with squares of muslin so that you don't lose half of your harvest in the nooks and crannies of the basket. Flowers are ready for storing when they have retained their colour but are considerably smaller – unlike leaves, they rarely dry to the point where they can be easily broken. In order to enjoy the flowers year-round, store them in glass jars, out of direct sunlight, carefully labelled with their English and Latin names. For the best possible perfume retention, dry them away from any direct heat, as heat and sunlight will evaporate off the volatile oils that cause the fragrance.

Medicine making

Infused oils and balms

One important thing to remember when making infused oils or balms in the spring, particularly if you will be using flowers, is that water will often lurk between petals and in the creases of flowers and leaves. Try, where possible, to pick dry flowers and leaves, but if this really isn't feasible, don't despair – you can use a dehydrator to partially dry your plant matter prior to medicine making. Alternatively, simply make the oil as you would normally; once the infusion is finished, decant the oil through kitchen paper into a clean Pyrex glass jug, preferably a clear one, and let it sit for at least two days. In many cases you will find that any water content in the oil will sink, and you can pour off the clean oil and throw away the murky stuff at the bottom. The same applies to leaf oils. It is important not to bottle murky oil, as this will send the whole batch rancid. The only possible exception to this rule is oil made from chickweed: I have often found that chickweed oil stays stubbornly cloudy and yet will, despite this, remain stable for quite a number of months. The best oils for medicine making, I have found, are organic seed oils, like sunflower, mainly because they are more stable. Sweet almond is lovely but expensive, and will often go rancid quite quickly. It is perhaps better suited to the making of skin creams and more delicate cosmetic and skin-care products.

As the drying season often really doesn't get off to a good start until late April, it is important to get to grips with some of the multitude of other ways in which you can use and store your spring herbs. Here are a few suggestions for you to try.

Infused wine, brandy, or vinegar

Herbs infuse very readily into all sorts of liquid mediums. Indeed, Culpeper often prescribed herbs digested in wine as a useful way of carrying their virtues, which is well worth remembering today and is certainly a precursor to our considerably stronger tinctures. If you are going to make medicinal wine, it is a good idea to let the herbs dry overnight first, as most wines don't have a particularly high alcohol content. With wines, spirits, or vinegars, try to use mostly surface-dry plants – they don't need to be bone dry, but use a clean, dry cloth to absorb the worst of the water on them.

Infusions in spirits, or tinctures, will last quite a considerable amount of time, whereas infusions in wine will need to be drunk fairly quickly, or they will turn to vinegar. If this happens, don't get rid of them: consider using them in salad dressings, as ingredients in cookery, or as topical applications. Vinegar infusions tend to be a great deal more stable.

If you choose to buy a tincture, this will be specified as a ratio followed by a percentage, such as 1:3 40%; the ratio signifies that 3 ml of liquid contains 1 g of the herb, and 40% indicates the percentage of alcohol in the liquid.

Decoctions and infusions

Straight-up infusions can be made and then either drunk, added to bath water or frozen in ice-cube trays. Short-term decoctions can be made by boiling the herb in water until the quantity has reduced by half, then either taking smaller doses of it throughout the day or freezing it in ice-cube trays. Long decoctions often don't need to be stored in the freezer. These are made by finely chopping whichever herbs or roots you want to preserve and boiling them up in plenty of water – assume 570 ml (20 fl oz) of water to 2–3 tbsp (30–45 g) of chopped herbs, topping the water level back up as it reduces down, and keeping the whole lot simmering for up to 4 hours. After 4 hours, simmer without topping up until the quantity has reduced down by at least a half – by this point you will sometimes notice an almost petrol-like skin on top of the water. I've certainly noticed this when I've made nettle long decoction – it gained a rainbow iridescence on the top of the inky coloured decoction, and the whole thing lasted months out of the fridge. Long decoctions can be taken in tablespoon doses, and can be rather fun to make, especially if the idea of cackling over potions appeals to you – it certainly does to me!

Freezing herbs

Those more delicate spring plants that really don't dry down well can be frozen for storage. Gather the herbs when they are at their best, make sure they are clean, then finely chop them and pack them into ice-cube trays. Put them in the freezer, and once they have fully frozen, you can put them into jars or boxes with labels on, and simply remove a cube when you need one.

Spring herbs for the medicine garden

Many of the herbs found in spring tend to be wild, so if you can possibly manage it, it can be a wonderful idea to have a little corner of your garden that you plant up with wildflowers, leaving gaps for some of our native plants to self sow. You never know which beautiful and useful plants may pop up, given room and a quiet invitation! Here are a few of my favourite wild plants found in the spring, with a very brief introduction to what you can use them for. Longer and more detailed articles on each are found throughout this book, along with some recipes and instructions for use.

Violet (*Viola odorata*) – flowering twice a year, in April and often again in October, pretty violet gives delicate and tasty flowers in the spring, which can be used along with the leaves to cool an over-hot disposition, acting on the lungs, digestive system, and nervous system – a very useful multi-purpose remedy.

Cowslips (*Primula veris*) and **primroses** (*P. versicolor*) – these pretty plants provide a plethora of sunny yellow flowers. If the weather permits, primrose will often begin flowering in late January or early February; the flowers can be picked and eaten or added to salads. Cowslips flower from April through to late May and give apricot-flavoured flowers that make a delicious snack. Medicinally, both plants act as a sedative, with benefits for anxiety, headaches and insomnia, and, additionally, with actions on the lungs and circulatory system.

Hawthorn (*Crataegus monogyna* / *C. laevigata*) – flowering in May and traditionally signalling the end of spring and the beginning of summer, hawthorn's scented flowers are a wonderful circulatory system tonic as well as being gently relaxing. This lovely tree is a common hedgerow plant in the UK, and there are quite a few varieties, all of which are used in a similar fashion. (For full details on hawthorn, see *Wild Medicine: Autumn and Winter.*)

Chickweed (*Stellaria media*) – providing both an edible salad plant and a medicine for lymph, skin, liver and kidneys, chickweed is a more difficult plant to grow, but if you leave space, there's a good chance she will show up and provide you with a juicy green patch of leaves that can be used both as food and for making medicine. Chickweed likes to grow in disturbed soil and often sneaks into my raised vegetable beds alongside the kale and the spinach.

Birch (*Betula pendula*) – growing quite happily in a large pot, birch will give you a huge yield of tender green leaves within a year or two of planting, providing medicine for a wide variety of ills. If you have space, you can always plant birch direct into the ground, and it will grow into a slender, elegant tree.

Herb robert (*Geranium robertianum*) – also known as stinky bob because of the fragrance of the leaves, herb robert often pops up where he is least expected, giving swathes of ferny green and red foliage and a fantastic array of mauve flowers. Herb robert is a wonderful wound healer, making really useful balms when combined with plantain, and also has a range of medicinal uses internally.

Plantain (*Plantago lanceolata*) – sometimes found in the wildflower section at garden centres, plantain grows readily in the grass and in verges and by the wayside. A great member of the medicine garden, this wonderful little plant will heal all sorts of skin wounds, cuts, grazes, bites and stings, as well as providing internal soothing of lung issues, stomach problems, and sinus- and head-cold-related discomforts.

Ground ivy (*Glechoma hederacea*) – another of the wild plants, this dainty little member of the mint family provides a great ground cover, so if you want to keep cleavers to a manageable number, this can be a great one to plant. Ground ivy also provides topical treatment for a variety of conditions; and it can be taken internally to improve the digestion and boost lung health, aiding and improving a wide range of lung issues including hayfever, bronchitis and repeated chest infections.

Birch
Betula pendula

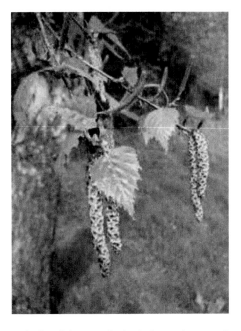

Also known as: lady of the woods, birk (Scandinavian)

Family   Betulaceae.

Habitat and description   Birch trees are a familiar sight in many countries around Europe. In the UK, they populate woodlands and gardens alike and are a glorious sight in the spring, when adorned with the first new green haze of growth – it is one of the first trees to noticeably leaf out. The bark is a shimmering silver colour with black textured areas and it peels easily from the trunk – in birch woods you can often find chunks of it adorning the ground. Many of the names given to it in different countries link back to a root word meaning "to shine" – not at all surprising, considering how beautifully silver the bark is. The twigs are a dark purple brown, with buds that begin a rich ochre brown when tightly closed but, as they loosen and begin to open, turn the luminous green we so love in the spring.

Birch grows to a height of roughly 25 m (80 ft), given the right circumstances; but generally it is not very long-lived, often rotting from the inside out as it ages. It is a very rapid-growing tree, often the outrider of slower-growing trees, which it protects as they grow. It is much beloved of fungi, from the tinder polypore to the famous chaga found in more northern climates, and turkey tail found all over the UK and Europe, all of which are either useful or medicinal or both, utilising the tree's salicylates in the production of their own healing compounds. The tree produces both male and female

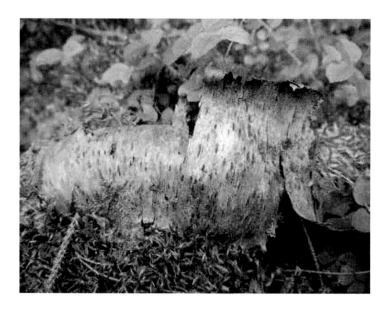

catkins, often on the same branch. The leaves are roughly spear-shaped, with toothed edges and a pointed tip; they are brilliant green in summer, aging to a rich gold in the autumn. A graceful birch tree leafed out in gorgeous golden colours with its strikingly silver bark in the autumn is a beautiful sight to see, especially when planted in profusion.

Where to find it   Birch is found in most of Europe (including Norway, Sweden and Finland and the UK), as well as in North America and Asia. Each country has its own native versions of the birch tree, which are especially adapted to cope with the soil and climate of its homeland, and many of these have medicinal uses.

Parts used   Leaves and bark are the most often used parts, with birch sap also being tapped in early spring to make into wines and syrups.

When to gather   Supple birch trees begin to produce tiny new leaves and catkins surprisingly early in the year, a welcome first indication of the arrival of spring. There are different schools of thought about the right time of year to have a go at tapping your birch tree – most agree late February to early March is a good time, as the tiny new leaves often begin to appear by late February, indicating that the sap has now risen high enough to invigorate the tree. The young leaves can be gathered once they are longer than 2.5 cm (1 in) – any smaller than this and I think it can be a bit difficult to get enough for medicine making, though a different school of plant medicine known as gemmology uses the buds specifically and would most likely pick them at the smaller stage.

If you are stripping the bark from the young twigs, snip off the smaller twigs – try to pick ones that will help thin out an overladen branch, or remove ones that are perhaps blocking a path, rather than removing bark from the trunk itself or from larger branches. Of course, if you have a birch that needs a bit more than basic cosmetic help, you're in luck! The bark can be shaved off in strips, keeping as much of the inner pith as you can, and dried in shallow baskets or in a dehydrator at a low heat. Store the dried bark pieces in dark glass jars, or use them fresh to tincture, if possible. Remember when stripping bark from trees never to ring it, as this will kill the tree – this is why I prefer to gather smaller twigs and branches if possible.

Medicines to make   Birch can be used to make a leaf-and-twig tincture; birch sap syrup can be made by boiling the tapped-off sap until the quantity reduces right down; birch elixir can be made with brandy; birch syrup can be made with the young leaves and twigs; or a birch leaf salve can be prepared by infusing the leaves in oil and adding beeswax. I like to gather the young leaves on a dry day and arrange them in wide baskets, turning the leaves over by flicking the basket lightly in the air.

Constituents   Betulinic acid, which is an anti-tumour agent; flavonoids; monoterpene glucosides; saponins; anthocyanins and volatile oils; salicylic acid.

Planetary influence   Venus.

Associated deities and heroes   Brighid, Thor, many of the Earth Goddesses, Frigga, and very probably many of the Mother Goddesses from around the world. Birch and its related trees are found in many different countries and many have their own links with local deities and folklore.

Festival   Imbolc, at the beginning of February.

Constitution   Cool and dry.

Actions and indications   Birch has long been used as an anti-inflammatory and alterative herb for the treatment of rheumatism and arthritis. The leaves, which are astringent and rather bitter to the taste, are often used to treat bladder and kidney infections such as cystitis. They are also rather laxative, so, when picked early in the season when they are just opening, they can be dried to make a tonic laxative to relieve simple constipation. I'd be inclined to suggest that this is especially useful when constipation has been caused by a lack of tone to the bowel muscles – the astringent properties of birch tone up the bowel walls nicely, and the herb, being cooling, is very good when mucous membranes have become over-excited and irritated. Consider combining it with a moistening and soothing mucous membrane tonic for this purpose, such as plantain leaf (*Plantago lanceolata* or *P. major*).

Due to its strong astringent components, the tea can also be used to relieve issues with the mouth, such as sores and bleeding gums – either drink the tea or use a strong tea or decoction as a mouthwash several times a day until relief is obtained. As a sedative, anodyne, and lymphatic agent, it can be used to ease the discomfort of sore muscles and relieve the water retention linked with ailments such as lymphoedema, which is linked with cellulitis. According to some sources, it can also be used to relieve gout, but given that gout often doesn't do too well with salicylic acid, be a little cautious with this use.

Birch leaves, drunk as a tea while young, also have a reputation for helping the body break down and expel gravel in the bladder or kidneys. It is high in potassium, so can help regulate and support correct water levels within the body's cells.

As an alternative, the young leaves can be tinctured in vodka in order to benefit liver and gall bladder function and relieve stomach ulcers, colds, and rheumatic conditions – all in all, a really useful addition to your home dispensary!

Externally the young leaves can be used to improve a wide variety of skin conditions, such as eczema and psoriasis. Boil up the leaves and twigs and add the cooled and strained liquid to the bathwater, or use it as a topical wash.

Folklore   Birch has long been the tree of new beginnings: a pioneer that will venture first onto disturbed earth, rendering it suitable for other plant and tree species to inhabit. It is one of the most sacred trees in Scandinavian folklore, being, in some schools of thought, the World Tree itself, and a ladder to the other realms. Fly agaric is most often found at the base of birch trees, and as a result this fungus is itself the source of much folklore. Birch is also found as part of the Ogham alphabet, itself a source of great mystery and controversy, where the tree symbolizes fresh starts, birth and rebirth.

Dose   One tsp (5 g), heaped, of the young leaves or freshly peeled bark to a cup of hot water, drunk up to three times a day. Tincture dosage – 3 ml of a cottage tincture in approximately 38% proof alcohol up to four times a day, as needed.

Contraindications   The young leaves contain salicylates, so if you are allergic to aspirin, do not use birch. Salicylic acid and gout do not usually play well together either, so for this condition use birch cautiously, if at all.

Birch recipes

Birch infused oil

Ingredients
- » 1 pint of loosely packed, freshly picked dry birch leaves
- » organic seed oil

Instructions   Check over the leaves for livestock and any damp bits – discard any insect-marked or discoloured leaves. Use a clean, dry cloth to mop up any water, as gathering herbs for oil making in the spring can be difficult with the amount of rain we get in the UK! If you have a few damp leaves, I suggest wiping them off as much as you can, then laying them out in a basket in a warm, dry place for a few hours to get the last bit to evaporate off. One easy way to dry the leaves is to lay out a clean, dry tea towel, lay out a single layer of the leaves, then place another tea towel over the top and pat it down using gentle but firm motions, making sure you cover the whole tea towel. Once you are sure the leaves are all dry, use a mezzaluna (a semi-circular chopping tool) or even a food processor to finely chop them, and pile them into the top of a double boiler.

Cover the herbs with the vegetable or seed oil, allowing ½ cm of oil on top and, making sure there is water in the bottom of the pot, put them on a low-to-moderate heat for at least an hour, keeping an eye on the water level to make sure it doesn't boil dry. By the time an hour has gone by, the oil should have turned a deep green colour, at which point the herbs can be filtered out. You can make a double-infused batch if you want to, by gathering and chopping a second batch of leaves and repeating the process, using the already infused oil instead of fresh. If you have a wood-burning stove, this is a lovely way to make the oil, as you will warm your home at the same time.

You can also make this infused oil in a slow cooker – just make sure it is on the low setting and leave it to infuse for at least 4 hours, or longer if possible. If you have any concerns about the possible presence of water in your finished oil, stand it overnight in a Pyrex jug or bowl. You will find that any water in the finished product will have sunk to the bottom, and you can pour off the oil and discard the water.

Birch salve

Ingredients

» 100 ml (3½ fl oz) of infused birch oil, as per recipe above
» 12 g of beeswax per 100 ml (3½ fl oz) of oil – beeswax pellets work well
» essential oils, as preferred: mint works beautifully here, as does orange – if you go for these two, use 10 drops of orange and 5 drops of mint per 100 ml (3½ fl oz)

Instructions   Pour the infused oil and the beeswax into the top of the clean, dry double boiler and put the whole thing on to warm through gently, stirring occasionally. Once the beeswax pellets have melted, stir it again thoroughly and add the essential oils. Up to 15 drops of essential oil per 100 ml (3½ fl oz) of oil makes for a pleasant, not overpowering fragrance. Stir the mixture again briefly and pour it into clean, dry jars, putting the lid on once the salve has cooled slightly. I like to rest the lid on as soon as the salves have been poured, to stop too much of the fragrance from evaporating off.

Birch salve and infused oil are both wonderful for cellulitis and for any conditions where muscles and joints are sore and inflamed – rheumatism, arthritis, sports injuries and strained muscles, for example. You can smear a generous layer of birch salve onto a clean cloth and bandage it lightly over a painful joint or muscle to really allow the salve to soak in steadily.

Birch tea or decoction with fresh leaves

Ingredients
- » 1 tsp, heaped, of fresh leaves per mug of water
- » 1 mug of water per person

Instructions   To make birch tea, first check over the birch leaves for marks or bugs, then finely chop them and put them into a teapot, cafetiere or tea ball before pouring over one mug of just-off-the-boil water per spoonful of leaves. Allow this mixture to steep for 5 minutes before drinking. You can add a slice of lemon, a pinch of cinnamon, or a dollop of honey to flavour it.

To make a decoction version of this, add 2 tbsp, heaped, of the chopped leaves per pint of water; you can also include smaller twigs, finely chopped. Put the whole lot into a saucepan on a moderate heat and simmer for 10 minutes, until reduced down by a third, then strain the liquid off. Store it in a bottle in the fridge – this will keep for three days.

Birch tea can be used internally to relieve gravel in the kidneys and bladder, ease sore muscles and rheumatic discomfort, and encourage excess water out of the system. For sore muscles, I'd suggest backing it up with the liberal application of the salve mentioned above. The tea can be drunk by the cupful, up to three times a day. The decoction can be drunk twice a day, by the half-cupful. Alternatively, you can use it as a bath or skin wash, or as a mouthwash. Topically the infusion or decoction can be used to relieve eczema, psoriasis and other itchy, inflamed skin conditions.

Birch tincture

Ingredients
- » 1 pint, at least, of loosely packed fresh birch leaves and young twigs
- » 1 bottle of vodka or brandy – basic supermarket own brands work just fine, but get the strongest one you can find

Instructions   As with the tea and oil recipes, check over the leaves and small twigs carefully. It doesn't matter if the surfaces are a little damp, as they will be covered in vodka. Using a sharp knife or mezzaluna, cut the leaves into small pieces – 5 mm square or smaller works well. The larger the surface area exposed to the alcohol, the more of the beneficial properties of the birch leaves will be preserved. If the twigs are really soft, you can also chop them with the mezzaluna or with a pair of kitchen scissors. If you use scissors, I suggest holding them right over the jar they will be put into, as they have a tendency to ping all over the place otherwise and you'll still find them in corners and under counters six months later! Pack the chopped leaves and twigs into a Kilner jar and pour over enough vodka to cover them, plus an extra 2.5 cm (1 in) depth of vodka on top. Put the lid on, shake it up thoroughly, then put it into a cool, dark place. Every couple of days, shake up the tincture to make sure the vodka covers all the plant matter, and if you need to, press the herbs back down under the level of the alcohol afterwards.

Leave the tincture to steep for a minimum of two weeks – I've had some steep for months, and that works just as well, so don't panic if you forget about it! When you are happy the tincture is strong enough, strain out the herbs and put the liquid back into a glass bottle. Remember to label the bottle carefully with the English and Latin names of your tincture, plus the date when it was made; also note down the strength of the alcohol originally used. The water content in the herbs will dilute it somewhat, but this should at least give you a rough idea of how long your tincture will last. As a rule of thumb, a tincture needs to be at least 20% alcohol to keep for long periods of time – less than this, and it will need to be used within a year.

Birch tincture can be used for relieving sore and inflamed muscles and as a gentle painkiller: 5–10 ml up to four times a day can work well, but start off with a small dose of just one teaspoon, and work up from there. It can also be used as a gentle liver and gallbladder tonic for those prone to sluggish liver function, perhaps in part where its use as a laxative for the relief of constipation also originates. Topically, you can apply it as a liniment to sore muscles, and rub it well in – this will also pull blood to the area, which can be as effective as the pain-killing properties of the tincture.

Birch elixir

Ingredients
- » 1 pint, at least, of fresh young birch leaves and twigs, finely chopped
- » brandy or vodka
- » local honey

Instructions   As with the tincture, pack the chopped leaves and twigs into a Kilner jar and pour over the alcohol, but make sure you also add at least 2 tbsp (approximately 30 g) of local honey. Pop the lid on and shake it up, then leave it to steep for the same length of time as you would a tincture. This sweeter-flavoured remedy can be more palatable and is used in much the same way as the tincture for internal use; it is not used externally, as it is rather sticky.

Birch honegar and vinegar

Ingredients
- » 1 pint of loosely packed birch leaves and young twigs, finely chopped
- » unpasteurised cider vinegar, with the mother still in
- » local honey

Instructions   Pile the chopped leaves and twigs into a Kilner jar and pour over the cider vinegar, adding at least 2 tbsp of local honey (30 g), as with the elixir method. Pop the lid on and shake it up, then leave it to steep for at least a month.

Once it has steeped for long enough, strain out the herbs and use as you would a regular cider vinegar. Add a tablespoon to a cup of cool water and sip to relieve constipation and ease sore joints.

If you want to use this topically, for skin rashes, bites and itchy complaints, leave out the honey and make a basic birch infused vinegar. This can be diluted 50/50 with water (birch water, if you happen to have tapped your tree, or use filtered tap water, or spring or rain water). The resulting liquid can be dabbed gently onto inflamed, hot, irritated skin to relieve and tone the skin, or put into a spray bottle and sprayed over the affected area.

Chickweed
Stellaria media

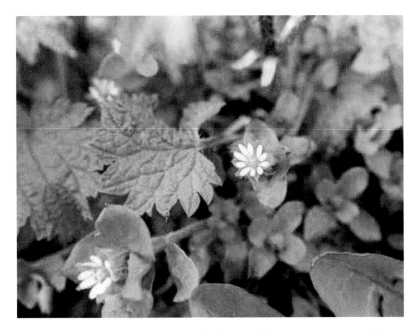

Also known as: bird's eye, cluckenweed, tongue grass, satinflower, winterweed, starweed, starwort

Family   Caryophyllaceae.

Habitat and description   Chickweed is an easily found annual growing all across Europe. It is one of our earlier medicinal plants to pop up in the spring, and can sometimes be found in February if the winter has been mild enough, straggling its way across beds and under hedges. The stems and leaves are juicy, pale green, and often low-growing, with oval-shaped opposite-paired leaves creeping their way up a stem that is smooth but for a single line of fine white hairs that grow up one side only. The tiny white flowers that give the plant its name of Stellaria resemble tiny star-like daisies – most enchanting when you look closely at them – and bloom at the axis of the upper leaf pairs throughout the spring, summer and autumn. This is one of those useful little plants that, if allowed to go to seed, will keep popping back up over and over again, so if you have a patch in your vegetable garden, let a little of it go to seed while you keep cutting and using the rest. You will almost certainly find that you have a second crop near the end of summer and early autumn that way.

Where to find it   Europe and much of North America, as well as most of Asia.

Parts used   Aerial parts (leaves and flowers) – the top 5 cm (2 in) are the tastiest bit for eating and can be quite easily picked between thumb and forefinger for adding to salads.

When to gather   Chickweed can be gathered from February until May, and often again later on in the year, though it goes a little leggy and stringy in the summer. The aerial parts can be

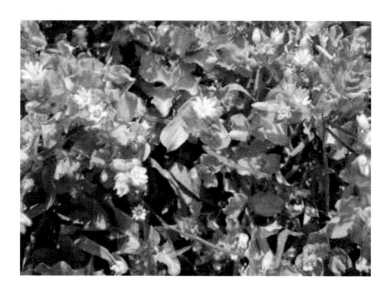

picked year-round for making infusions, skin washes, balms, infused oils and tinctures, but if you tincture it, remember that it is only good for one year, after which you will need to make a fresh batch.

Medicines to make Chickweed can be added to soups, stews, pestos, and any other recipe that calls for spring greens; it is best gathered in spring for this purpose, as later on it becomes a little leggy and less tender. It can also be lightly steamed as a side vegetable, if you pick the top few centimetres only, and the best part of it is that it will grow back again if you do this – a bit like giving a chive plant a haircut, really! This is one of those herbs that really benefits from a water or oil method of preparation, and to get the very best out of those soothing mucilage properties, consider a cold water preparation. That way you don't risk any of those delicate properties breaking down through the use of heat.

You can make larger quantities of chickweed infusion to put in a bath to soothe skin issues such as eczema and psoriasis, as well as chickenpox. Or juice the plant and add a small amount of the juice to smoothies and shakes to really help the lymph system do its job well, and by extension to really benefit the joints and musculoskeletal system. I like to gather the flowering tops on a dry day and infuse them in oil twice to make a lovely healing skin salve for after sunburn and to relieve cuts and grazes, though this is not so suitable for eczema and psoriasis. Try a gentle skin wash instead for these conditions, as they are better off without being covered with oils that stop the skin from breathing naturally.

Constituents Flavonoids, including rutin, phenolic acids, trace amounts of copper, coumarins, saponin glycosides, vitamin C.

Planetary influence Moon.

Associated deities and heroes Maiden Goddesses, Brigantia.

Festival Personally I usually associate this plant with Imbolc.

Constitution   Cool and moist.

Actions and indications   As a cooling, soothing herb, chickweed has a number of indications for skin problems, used both internally and externally. Taken internally as a lymphatic agent, it improves the flow and drainage of lymph around the body and can, as a result, improve rheumatism and arthritis and other inflammatory conditions resulting in water retention, as well as skin problems such as acne, pruritis (itching), eczema and psoriasis.

Fresh chickweed stems, leaves and flowers can be chopped and bashed in the mortar and pestle to make a poultice for inflamed, sore joints that is helpful for problems such as gout, where it can help to draw out some of the heat that causes such intense pain. This poultice can also be used to remove grit or dirt from wounds and for boils and abscesses: the mucilage component can draw out the trapped poison that has caused the problem in the first place. In fact, this herb is so cooling and soothing that it can be used to ease and benefit any condition resulting in hot, inflamed skin or mucous membranes, as well as internal inflammation. As an alterative, it balances water levels throughout the body and is an all-round tonic for the whole body, with particular benefit for the kidneys. An old traditional use was as a weight-loss herb, which could certainly be believed as it does help to regulate water retention and helps the body to break down and remove fat deposits.

Use the herb to make a wonderful cream for skin problems such as eczema and psoriasis, though bear in mind wet forms of psoriasis need to breathe. A strong tea or juice of chickweed can be used to relieve minor burns and sunburn and as a wash for itchy, inflamed skin problems such as chickenpox. A salve of chickweed can be used to make a drawing poultice for splinters and abscesses, handy for year-round usage.

Drunk as a really strong tea, it can be used to relieve constipation that has been caused by drying out of the system, as it restores moisture and softens the stool enough to allow easier passage from the body.

Folklore   Chickweed has long been used as a favoured food for pets, including chickens and other birds, rabbits, guinea pigs and others. It also makes a great food for humans – the vitamin C content boosts the system in spring, kicking it back into active life. Enjoy it in soups with nettles, as a juice added to smoothies or as a green salad leaf or vegetable in its own right.

Dose   Fresh as a vegetable, whenever you fancy it. As a tea, 1 tsp, heaped, of fresh or dried herb to a cup of hot water drunk up to three times a day. A cold infusion would work very well to preserve the softening, soothing aspects of the herb, and if you use this method, enjoy a mug or two of it a day, or freeze it in ice-cube trays so you can still enjoy it later in the summer once the plant has begun to get a little stringy.

Contraindications   Can precipitate a healing crisis when treating psoriasis, eczema and acne: while the body is driving out the cause of these issues, the conditions themselves get worse before they get better. If this happens, drop the dose right back for a week or two and gradually increase it over a fortnight.

Chickweed recipes

Chickweed salve

Ingredients
- » 1 pint, loosely packed, of chickweed, fresh from the garden but dry – no surface water like rain or dew
- » organic seed or vegetable oil
- » beeswax (you can use jojoba or almond wax if you prefer but they don't tend to set very well)
- » lavender or chamomile essential oil

Instructions   Make sure your chickweed is free of bugs or bird poop, then chop it thoroughly, as finely as you can. I would also recommend putting the whole lot into a mortar and pestle and giving it a really good bash once it has been chopped, just to really get the sap flowing. Transfer it into the top of a double boiler, and cover it with the oil, until you can see a thin sheen of oil on top of the herbs. Put the double boiler on to simmer, and allow the whole lot to infuse for at least 20 minutes – longer is better. Once the oil has turned a rich green, take it off the heat and pour it through a jelly bag into a jug. Let the oil settle for at least half an hour, to allow any water to sink to the bottom, then carefully pour off the oil from the top, leaving the water behind – that way you can avoid using the water content, which could potentially turn the oil rancid. Allow 12 g of beeswax per 100 ml (3½ fl oz) of oil, and warm the two ingredients in the double boiler until the beeswax melts. Add the essential oils – about 10 drops of lavender or 5 drops of chamomile per 100 ml (3½ fl oz) of oil works well to make a lovely soothing salve. Stir the essential oils in briefly, then pour the salve into clean jars.

This salve is superb for any itchy skin issues, especially insect bites and stings, and can also promote the healing of scrapes and minor cuts. It keeps for a long time, and does not need to be stored in the fridge, as long as it is kept out of direct sunlight and the murky stuff at the bottom of the oil mix wasn't added to the salve. A note about the oil component – I often find that this oil ends up a little on the murky side, but I have also noticed that, more often than not, it will store just fine and will not go rancid. So don't panic if your oil doesn't come out as clear as you would like, for all is not lost! If the oil is cloudy, I recommend leaving it in a glass bowl or Pyrex jug for a few days to see if the moisture content will settle. If at the end of three days it is still cloudy, you should find that it will be fairly stable and can be stored, in a cool, dark cupboard for up to a year.

Chickweed juice

Ingredients
  » plenty of chickweed
  » 1–2 tbsp (15–30 ml) of water

Instructions   The chickweed stems need to be cut into pieces no longer than 5 cm (2 in) before you pile them into a food processor. Blitz in short, 30-second pulses until the mixture has formed a juicy green pulp, then add 1 tbsp (15 ml) of water, and blitz it again. I find the addition of a small amount of water loosens up the mixture and makes it easier to squeeze it out through a piece of muslin. If the chickweed mix hasn't turned into a proper green pulp in the bottom of the food processor, add a little more water and blitz it again. Finally, line a sieve over a large bowl with a piece of clean muslin and tip the chickweed into it, using a silicone spatula to scrape out the bowl thoroughly. Gather up the sides of the muslin and squeeze the chickweed thoroughly to extract as much juice as possible. By the time you are done, you should have a dark emerald-green liquid in the bottom of the bowl, and the chickweed itself should have been reduced to a small, well-squeezed pile of green leaf matter, which can either be frozen to use as a poultice later on, or composted.

The juice can be added to smoothies and glasses of water, or applied directly to sore, inflamed skin. In the case of eczema or weeping psoriasis, consider mixing it with a little chamomile aromatic water and putting it into a spray bottle that you can spray directly onto the affected area.

Chickweed infusion

Ingredients
- » a handful of chickweed
- » water off the boil

Instructions   A basic infusion of chickweed is very simple to make, with the added benefit that it takes only a few minutes. Just chop the herbs finely, put them into a teapot or cafetiere, then pour over enough just-off-the-boil water to make a cup of infusion. I allow 1 tsp, heaped, of chopped fresh herbs to one mug of water. As a straight infusion, drink a cup up to three times a day, to reduce water retention, relieve rheumatism and arthritis, and encourage the body to break down fatty deposits.

To make a herbal bath, I suggest allowing 2 tbsp (30 g) of chopped fresh herb to 570 ml (20 fl oz) of water and letting it steep until it is cool before straining out the herbs and adding the resulting liquid to the bathwater, or use a cotton wool pad soaked in the liquid to gently bathe itchy, sore parts of the body.

Chickweed cold infusion

Ingredients
- » 1 tsp, heaped, of chickweed
- » cold water

Instructions   Like the basic infusion, cold infusions are also really simple to make, but they do need to be planned in advance. Just check over your chickweed, chop the fresh plant matter, and allow 1 tsp, heaped, (5 g) to a cup of water. Put it into a Kilner jar, top it up with cold water, allowing effectively one mug of cold water per teaspoon of herb, cover with a lid, and put it in the fridge overnight. A slow infusion like this results in little to no breakdown of the mucilage content, which is what makes the plant so soothing.

Cold infusions can be drunk to relieve rheumatism, gout and arthritis as well as to improve lymph flow, which may well benefit skin problems as well, or you could use it as a soothing skin wash for itchy, inflamed skin conditions.

A soothing chickweed skin cream

Ingredients
- » 125 ml (4½ fl oz) chickweed infused oil
- » 125 ml (4½ fl oz) lavender flower water or chickweed infusion or juice (see recipes above)
- » 12 g beeswax
- » 1 tsp (5 g) glycerine
- » 5 ml vitamin E oil
- » 5 drops German chamomile essential oil
- » 2 drops lavender essential oil (if desired)

Instructions Heat the infused oil and beeswax in the top of a bain marie over a pan of simmering water, until the beeswax melts. Gently warm the flower water and glycerine in a small pan. Pour the oil and wax mixture into a food processor and allow it to cool until it is no longer translucent, but not until it has set. Add the flower water and glycerine mix a little at a time, blending between each addition, until it has completely emulsified with the oil mixture. Add the vitamin E and the essential oils just before you pour the cream into jars, blending briefly to fold it into the cream. Store the finished cream in the fridge. This cream blend can be used for a variety of itchy skin conditions and can be applied as needed. Vegetable glycerine can be sourced from most cosmetic supply companies – go for an organic version if you possibly can.

You can also use a strong infusion of chickweed instead of lavender water for a pure chickweed cream for use on itchy skin, and use an oil blend that combines lavender, chickweed and chamomile infused oils. This cream can be applied multiple times throughout the day to relieve the itching and discomfort of insect bites and stings, burns and sunburn, as well as for minor cuts and grazes.

Chickweed in garlic butter

Ingredients

> » 1 good handful of chickweed tops, freshly picked and checked for livestock; these need to be gathered in early spring, as later on they do become rather stringy
> » one good dab of butter – around 10 g – is usually plenty
> » salt to taste
> » 1 large clove of organic garlic
> » a squeeze of lemon juice

Instructions   Put the butter into a frying pan and put it on a medium heat, to allow the butter to melt. Finely chop the garlic and add it to the pan, cooking it gently until translucent. While the butter slowly melts and coats the pan and the garlic cooks, pat your herbs dry if they are a bit damp, then roughly chop them and add them to the pan, stirring regularly to make sure they cook evenly and get a coating of the heated butter. Add a squeeze of lemon at the end, and sprinkle over some seasoning – herb salt works well, as does Himalayan salt with garlic or other herbs mixed into it. Serve as a side dish with fish or any other main meal or light lunch, or you could even top a slice of fresh bread with it.

Chickweed poultice

Ingredients / equipment
- » 1 large handful of fresh chickweed herb
- » a food processor or a mezzaluna, and some patience
- » a small amount of warm water
- » an old tea towel and a length of bandage

Instructions   Using either the food processor or the mezzaluna, chop the herbs as finely as you can manage – the finer the better, really! You can then pile the herbs into a mortar and add a tiny trickle of warm water before using the pestle to pound the herbs into a thick mush. Smear the thick green paste onto a clean tea towel and bandage it in place over boils, nasty bites and stings or sore or inflamed areas to ease pain, draw out toxins and encourage healing. Leave it on for between half an hour and half a day, depending on how inconvenient leaving it in place is. You can compost the spent herbs, and wash and reuse the tea towel and bandage.

Cleavers
Galium aparine

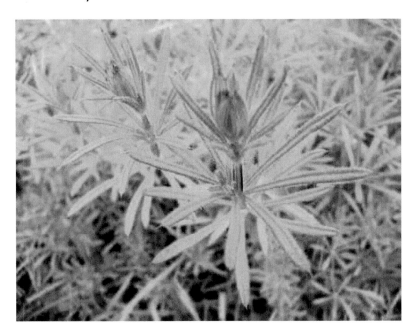

Also known as: goosegrass, burweed, goosebill, clivers, clives, catchweed, bed straw, little sweethearts, hayriff, robin-run-in-the-hedge, mutton chops, everlasting friendship, sticky buds, scratch-weed, grip-grass, eriffe, hedgeheriff, scratweed, love-man, barweed

Family   Rubiaceae.

Habitat and description   This sticky-leaved, pernicious explorer rampages quite happily through gardens, hedgerows, roadsides, wooded areas – anywhere there are places it can clamber up. It grows very readily in hedgerows, where it will scramble up in amongst the hawthorn, ash and elder and easily cover half the plants in a veil of pointed leaves. If you aren't careful, it will choke out other plants. It is actually quite pretty when it flowers – tiny, white four-petalled stars that are easily missed unless you look closely. The seeds are small, round and hard and will stick to anything they come into contact with – animal fur (especially that of dogs and cats, who seem to love to bring half the plant back inside with them!), clothes, hair, skin: you name it, they will stick to it.

The lanceolate leaves are arranged in whorls around the central stem, which is quite grooved and will climb or sprawl according to what support is available, covering hedges and taking over half the garden if given free rein. The seeds start out a rich green and dry to a medium brown; they have been used to make a coffee substitute. The whole fresh plant is a juicy green in colour, really vibrant and vivid in spring, when it is at its best, and fading to a slightly paler colour as the summer goes on. It is one of those plants that makes weeding quite good fun in the summer – you grab and pull what you think is one handful of the stems and before you know it, you've weeded half the garden and pulled up over five metres of the stuff.

Where to find it   Europe, parts of Asia and North Africa, as well as much of North and South America, Australia, New Zealand and Canada.

Parts used   In the spring, aerial parts – the top 25–35 cm (10–14 in) – are usually the best bits, as closer to the ground the plant becomes increasingly tough. The whole plant can be used as a pot herb, or steamed and eaten as a vegetable. In autumn the seeds can be dried and roasted to make a coffee substitute (which I freely admit I have yet to try – so far I haven't found anything that measures up to a good cup of coffee, but maybe I just haven't been willing to give up my caffeine addiction . . .). Apparently cleaver seed coffee tastes nearly as good as the real thing, so it could well be worth a try if you have the patience to gather up enough of the brown seeds. The roots produce a reddish dye, which can even tint the colour of bird bones, if they eat the roots.

When to gather   I like to gather my cleavers in the spring, from March through til May, as it is at its vibrant best then; this also offers the added bonus that the more you pull out now, the less you will have to deal with it taking over the garden later on!

Medicines to make   You can eat the very young plants in soups and stews or even as a lightly steamed salad vegetable, but you do need to use it for this purpose while young, as later in the season it really becomes too tough to be worth bothering with. Gather large handfuls to juice, infuse in oil, tincture or drink as a tea or decoction to relieve a wide variety of ailments.

Constituents   Iridoids, such as asperuloside and asperulosidic acid; polyphenolic acids, including gallic and caffeic acids, to

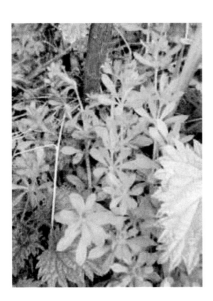

name but a few; alkaloids; flavonoids; anthraquinone derivatives predominantly in the roots.

Planetary influence   Moon.

Associated deities and heroes   None found at present, though given the plant's ability to twine around, up and over pretty much anything, maybe snake deities, who knows!

Festival   Ostara. Some also say the Autumn Equinox.

Constitution   Cool and moist.

Actions and indications   Cleavers are a well-known lymphatic tonic, making it an excellent addition to medicines to treat skin eruptions and related conditions as well as to get the lymph system moving. It can be used to treat any problems causing swollen, congested glands: add it to mixtures to treat colds that have caused swollen and painful lymph glands.

For the skin, the herb is fantastic for hormone-ridden teenagers, as it is excellent for clearing acne prone skin. It can also be used to treat eruptive skin conditions, such as psoriasis, eczema and boils, though for this purpose it is best used as a fresh plant extract. It is useful for the relief of the symptoms of childhood diseases such as mumps and chicken pox.

It can also be added to prescriptions for those suffering from painful urinary tract infections, as the plant is a soothing, anti-inflammatory diuretic, great for cystitis and related painful conditions such as urinary gravel, for bed-wetting in children, as well as for irritable bladder in all ages.

Because it is so beneficial for the lymph system, cleavers can also be a useful adjunct to cancer treatment, although again I would strongly recommend you see your local herbalist instead of self-medicating for this purpose. The herb seems to be specific particularly to breast and skin tumours.

The herb has a history of use for liver congestion and its related problems of nausea and jaundice, as well as to treat hepatitis. By extension, it could probably also be used to treat cirrhosis, and I recommend drinking it regularly in cases of fatty liver disease to help the body clear out the excess fat that has accumulated around the liver. This needs to be done alongside lifestyle changes.

It has also been used by some herbalists for nerve problems, though not having used it for this myself, I have no real stories to tell about it. Given the appearance of the seeds and the way the herb can climb anywhere it wants, there is a certain amount of Doctrine of Signatures linkage to both nerves and lymph nodes. The Doctrine of Signatures is an old method of assignment that gives medicinal virtues to plants based on the look of a plant, the colour of any flowers or seeds, the shape of leaves and other parts, and where and how it grows.

Topically, it can be used to make creams and washes to treat burns, skin infections and fresh wounds.

Cleavers is generally best used as a fresh plant extract, so pick it and tincture it fresh, or make a strong tea from it – though remember that if you tincture it fresh, you will find that the potency dies off after a year, as with chickweed, so you may find it beneficial to make a new batch every spring.

Folklore   The Anglo-Saxon nickname of "hedge-rife" referred to a tax collector or robber. The Greeks knew it as "philanthropon", from its tendency to cling to things. The ancient Greeks used to make a makeshift sieve, using cleavers, to filter milk through. It has also long been used for a similar purpose in Sweden, and in some parts is still used this way.

Dose   A tea can be made from 1 tsp, heaped, of the dried herb infused in hot water and drunk three times a day. A cold infusion can also be made and drunk regularly. Some give the dosage as 10 ml per single dose, others say drop doses. Personally, I would not use more than about 30 ml of tincture in a week's prescription unless I was using it for acute illness, predominantly due to the plant's ability to bring about a healing crisis in some people.

Contraindications   Be aware that, like chickweed, cleavers can cause a healing crisis, especially when dealing with skin disorders, so go carefully.

Cleavers recipes

Cleavers juice for eczema and psoriasis

Ingredients / equipment
» lots of fresh cleavers from the garden – the more the merrier!
» a blender
» a small amount of water just off the boil; you can probably omit the hot water if you happen to have one of those handy NutriBullet-type blenders

Instructions   Pick over the fresh cleavers and make sure it is free from livestock and bird poop, discarding any bits of leaf that have been chomped on or are soiled. Wash the leaves thoroughly under the cold tap, then chop roughly into 2.5 cm (1 in) long pieces and pack them into the blender. You do need to chop the herbs first – if you don't, they are likely to get tangled around the central pillar of the blender instead of getting minced. Add a small amount of water just off the boil: 2–3 tbsp (30–45 ml) to half a blender of herbs works well. Put the lid on and whizz the herbs until they have been reduced to a deep, rich, green, juicy pulp.

Put the pulp into a jelly cloth, a square of muslin, or a clean tea towel that has been rinsed through in boiling water to remove any fabric softener, then pull in the tops and squeeze the pulp as hard as you can to extract as much juice as possible. The resulting sap will be brilliant emerald green and smell like a spring morning after rain; it can be added to soups and stews, smoothies and teas, or a large glass of water, along with some lemon and ginger. Topically, you can use it to bathe irritated, sore skin, eczema and psoriasis, or to put into a warm bath to soothe skin infections and irritations such as chicken pox. If you have more juice than you can use, simply freeze it in ice-cube trays until you need it. You can take it out of the freezer and add it to pints of water on hot days, as a lovely way to get the herb into your system.

Cleavers infusion

Ingredients
- » small handful of fresh cleavers
- » water just off the boil

Instructions   The infusion is very simple to make. Just gather a small handful of fresh cleavers and finely chop them before you put them into a teapot. Cover the herbs with a mug of water just off the boil and let it steep for 5 minutes before you pour the resulting tea through a tea strainer. You can sweeten the tea with honey and add a slice of lemon if you want to, then drink it up to three times a day to improve lymph function and act as a gentle liver tonic.

Cleavers cold infusion

Ingredients
- » 2–3 25-cm (10-in.) pieces of cleavers
- » fresh spring water or filtered water
- » large glass jar with a lid

Instructions   Just bundle up the stems and give them a few twists in three or four places up the stem, to break the surface and encourage the juices to extract into the water properly. Put the stems into a large glass jar and pour over enough water to cover them, then put the lid on and put the jar into a fridge overnight. The next day you can pour off the water and drink it. Cleavers water has a delicate, greens and cucumber flavour that is very refreshing. Why not freeze some in ice cubes for adding to cold drinks or water later in the summer?

Cleavers cottage tincture

Ingredients
  » 1 pint, at least, of loosely packed fresh cleavers tops
  » vodka or brandy, as strong as you can afford

Instructions   Finely chop the fresh, clean cleavers, and pile them into a Kilner jar before you cover them with the alcohol, allowing an extra 2.5 cm (1 in) on top of the herbs. Pop the lid on and leave to infuse for at least a fortnight, shaking it up regularly to make sure the alcohol covers all the herbs properly. At the end of this time, filter it through a jelly cloth and bottle it. Take up to 10 ml three times a day to support the lymph system.

For an alcohol-free version of this, use cider vinegar instead – just replace the vodka or brandy with unpasteurised cider vinegar along with a dollop of honey, if you want it slightly sweetened, then drink it diluted with plenty of water. 10 ml of cider vinegar to 240 ml (8¾ fl oz) of water is usually pretty palatable. If you make this version without honey, you can also dilute it and use it as a skin wash for itchy, inflamed skin conditions.

Coltsfoot
Tussilago farfara

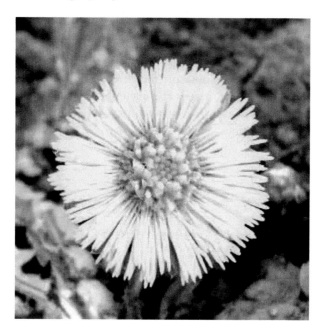

Also known as: horsehoof, foalswort, coughwort, donnhove, son-before-father, baccy plant

Family Asteraceae.

Habitat and description A welcome sight in February and March, coltsfoot's sunny flowers pop up and star the ground in thick clusters of yellow, well before the leaves make an appearance. The undersides of the flowers – and, indeed, the flower bud before it opens – is a vivid reddish yellow colour; the first young leaves start to appear before flowering has quite finished. Later in the season the flowers give way to silky white tufts of seeds that resemble superficially those of the dandelion, though upon closer inspection the texture is different as is the arrangement of the seeds themselves. The leaves are a distinctive shape, roughly hoof shaped with gently pointed spurs, softly downy undersides, and a thick, almost rubbery feeling when you bend them. They are a silvery green in colour and can be gathered from April onwards for making cough medicines; the flowers can be picked earlier and dried in baskets. The leaves begin small, no more than 2.5 cm (1 in) across; they can be up to 30 cm (12 in) across once they are fully grown. The very young leaves are covered with a silvery grey downy fuzz that rubs off as the leaves grow.

Coltsfoot prefers waste ground and will grow merrily along-side streams, between cracks in concrete and other places, preferring alkaline soil where possible. If you want to grow it in your garden, either put it in a wild area, where it can spread to its little heart's content, or plant it in a lovely big pot so that it won't take over your garden. Mine has now escaped its original location and is working hard to colonise the lawn.

Where to find it   Europe, Asia, North Africa and both North and South America.

Parts used   Flowers and leaves.

When to gather   Gather the flowers when they open from February to April, and the leaves later on, in April, May and June; dry them both before combining them. If the weather is very damp when you collect them, consider putting the herbs into a dehydrator, so that they can dry down properly.

Medicines to make   Coltsfoot is another herb with pyr-rolizidine alkaloid content, so those with impaired liver function must avoid using it. This is one of those herbs that is a medicine, not a tonic, so you really shouldn't need to use it over extended periods of time. It seems that the toxic alkaloids may not extract into water, only into alcohol, and for this reason I suggest the infusion method as the best way of taking this herb for short periods of time.

I like to make coltsfoot tea or syrup for chesty coughs and to help the body expel dust and particles that may be trapped in the lungs, for which it can be drunk twice a week at a dose of one or two cups a day maximum. Topically, an infused oil or salve can be handy.

Constituents   Tannins, mucilage, bitter glycosides, triterpenes, saponins, zinc, pyrollizidine alkaloids.

Planetary influence   Venus.

Associated deities and heroes   None known.

Festival   None known.

Constitution   Cool and balancing.

Actions and indications   Used as a poultice or salve, coltsfoot has a powerfully astringent, disinfectant and wound-healing effect, making it extremely useful for the healing of varicose veins, leg ulcers, bites and stings.

In addition to this, a strong tea can be used externally to

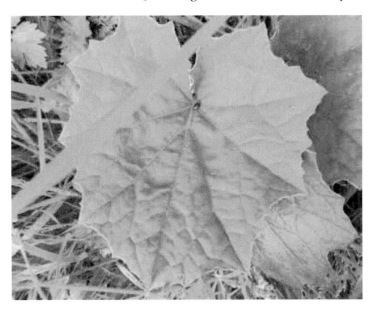

normalise oil secretions of the skin and hair, making it a great addition to the regime of anyone struggling with oil-related acne or dandruff. Just use it as a wipe for the skin or as a final rinse of the hair, making a fresh cup for this use every other day, or freeze strong coltsfoot tea in an ice-cube tray and defrost as needed.

Internally, coltsfoot can be used for acute and chronic bronchitis and whooping cough, as it softens irritation of the throat and relieves bronchial spasms while helping the body to cough up phlegm that has accumulated in the chest. It is particularly good at loosening stuck phlegm that cannot otherwise be removed. It has been used to reduce scarring from tuberculosis and emphysema, and according to some sources a single weekly dose can help the lungs cleanse themselves of pollution, making it very useful for those travelling in polluted atmospheres. I've certainly given it to my partner, a bladesmith, to help reduce irritation of the lungs after working with wood and metals, as even using a good mask, some particles can get through.

Coltsfoot can be used for asthma, as it thins mucus and relieves bronchial spasms, though it needs to be used in small doses for this as it can encourage too much expectoration too quickly. Start with teaspoons of the tea and work up from there. The same principle can be applied to using this herb for chronic bronchitis.

Folklore   There is very little folklore surrounding the humble coltsfoot. The name 'son before father' alludes to the plant's tendency to flower before the leaves appear. Much older forms of medicine held that the leaves must be burned on charcoal as part of a complicated cough remedy. Many of the folk names allude to the shape of the leaves, which seem to resemble that of a hoof.

Dose   Best used as a tea, so allow 1 tsp of the tea to a cup of hot water and steep for 5 minutes. Drink up to three times a day to relieve irritable coughs and encourage the body to remove excess phlegm. Start with a small dose at first, as it can lead to expectorating large amounts of phlegm very quickly! The tincture can also be used, but as the pyrrolizidine alkaloids extract in alcohol far more readily than in water, no more than 2 ml twice a day is recommended. The tea is considered safe, as the toxic alkaloids do not extract this way and are destroyed by boiling. If in doubt or with any concern about the alkaloids, or with a history of liver ill health, use alternative herbs instead.

Contraindications   Due to the presence of toxic alkaloids, albeit only in trace amounts, use as tea only, and for no more than two weeks at a time. It must be avoided by anyone whose liver function is impaired. If you are going to use a tincture, only use this for short periods of time: after about three days, consider using plantain leaf instead.

Coltsfoot recipes

Coltsfoot and plantain syrup

Ingredients
- » 1 handful each of fresh plantain and coltsfoot
- » 1 stem of mint for flavouring
- » thyme: 2 tbsp (approximately 15 g) of the fresh herb, if you have some handy, or 1 tbsp (10 g) of dried herb
- » 570 ml (20 fl oz) of water
- » 500 g (1 lb 1½ oz) brown unrefined sugar

Instructions   Check all of the fresh herbs for unexpected livestock, and rinse if necessary. Discard any yellowing or bird-fouled leaves, and then chop the herbs finely. This is quite easy to do if you tear them up by hand first into smaller pieces, then either chop them with a mezzaluna or sharp knife, or put them in a mortar and bash them with the pestle until the juices run. Do the same with the mint (leaves and stem) and the thyme, then put the whole lot into a pan with the water. Bring the concoction to a steady simmer and allow it to cook for 10 minutes, stirring occasionally. Keep a lid on the mixture at this stage, as the volatile oils will evaporate off if you do not.

Strain out the herbs, pour in the sugar, then warm the concoction, stirring it until the sugar dissolves. Bring it to a boil and allow it to cook for 10 minutes, keeping an eye on it to make sure it doesn't stick on the bottom of the pan and burn. Take it off the heat and pour it into bottles while it is still hot, as this will ensure a good seal. A good dose of this for coughs and chest infections is 1–2 tsp of the syrup every couple of hours. This recipe will keep for a long while in the fridge – I've known it to keep for up to a year if the ratio of sugar to liquid is high enough.

You can, instead, make it with honey – chop the herbs finely, mash them thoroughly using a mortar and pestle, then stir the green pulp into a jar of runny honey. Leave the whole lot to steep for at least two weeks before using it. You can add this to herb teas if you wish, or take it as it is for coughs, as listed above. Keep this syrup in the fridge.

Coltsfoot salve

Ingredients
- » 1 pint of young coltsfoot leaves, picked on a dry day
- » organic seed or vegetable oil
- » beeswax pellets – 12 g for every 100 ml (3½ fl oz) of resulting oil
- » essential oil to scent, as preferred – consider mint, orange or lavender as possibilities

Instructions   As with all infused-oil recipes, check the leaves first to make sure there are no bugs, droppings or water on them, then finely chop them and put into the top of a double boiler, or alternatively pile them into a slow cooker and just cover them with the oil. If you are using a double boiler, make sure there is water in the bottom section, and let the oil and herbs steep over simmering water for at least an hour. These are fairly thick leaves, so I like to make sure they have plenty of time to infuse. If you are using a slow cooker, put the lid on and let them steep on a low to medium heat for at least four hours. Once you are happy with the colour of your oil, which should be turning green by the end, filter out the leaves. Repeat the process with a second set of leaves if you want to, to make a really strong infused oil.

To make the balm, measure out the oil and allow 12 g of beeswax for every 100 ml (3½ fl oz) of coltsfoot-infused oil. You don't have to turn all of your oil into balm if you don't want to – just bottle any you don't use, label it carefully with the name, date and some basic uses for it, and store it out of direct sunlight. For the balm, put the beeswax and oil into the top of a double boiler over a pan of simmering water and allow it to warm through until the wax has melted, stirring occasionally. Add up to 10 drops of essential oil for each 100 ml (3½ fl oz) of infused oil – mint can be a lovely one, or add lavender for an all-purpose mixture. Stir it briefly to make sure the scent is properly mixed with the balm, then pour it into clean, dry jars and rest the lid on top to stop the scent from evaporating off. Once cool, close the lids tightly and label. The balm can be stored in a cool, dry place; preferably not in a fridge, as this will make it set completely solid. It should last anywhere from six months to several years.

This balm is very useful topically for varicose veins, leg ulcers, bites and stings, and as a general-purpose wound healer for cuts and grazes, as it is antibacterial and astringent.

Coltsfoot poultice

Ingredients
- » at least 1 pint of coltsfoot leaves
- » small amount of water

Instructions   Coltsfoot poultices are very simple to make. You can either finely dice the fresh leaves, add a tiny bit of water, and mash them up using a mortar and pestle before bandaging them in place, or you can smear a generous amount of the balm (see previous recipe) onto a clean tea towel and bandage it firmly over the bothersome area. Make sure you don't cut off the blood supply! Leave it on for an hour, then remove and gently rinse away the excess if you have used fresh herbs. Coltsfoot balm can be rubbed into the skin afterwards. This can be a lovely way of soothing nasty stings and insect bites, as well as helping to tighten up varicose veins.

Coltsfoot tea

Ingredients
- » 2 tsp, heaped, of fresh coltsfoot leaves, or 1 tsp, heaped, of dry crumbled coltsfoot leaves
- » cup of hot water

Instructions   Put 1 tsp, heaped, of chopped dry leaves or 2 tsp, heaped, of fresh leaves and a cup of hot water into a teapot and let it infuse for 10 minutes, then strain and drink one cup up to twice a day to encourage expectoration and help the lungs clear themselves of toxins. Expect a lot more phlegm production after this tea, which is an attractive yellow-green colour and tastes surprisingly mild and sweet! You can also use this infusion as a skin wash for the face and hair, to restore oil balance.

Coltsfoot vinegar

Ingredients
- » ½ pint of loosely packed coltsfoot leaves
- » unpasteurised cider vinegar

Instructions   Finely chop the herbs and pack them into a Kilner jar, then pour over the unpasteurised cider vinegar until it covers the leaves, with an extra 1.25 cm (½ in) on top. Let the mixture steep for a fortnight, then filter out the herbs, bottle, and label the resulting vinegar. The best way to use this is combined with flower waters as a toner or as a scalp mask – proportions are entirely up to you. For really oily skin, you may want equal parts vinegar and aromatic water, but if the problem is only minor, dilute it down around 1 part vinegar to 8 parts aromatic water. Use it as a final hair rinse, or use a cotton wool pad to apply it to the face, neck, back and shoulders in the case of acne. This should dry it up nicely, reduce the redness and swelling and balance the skin pH as well as normalising skin oil production.

Cowslip
Primula veris

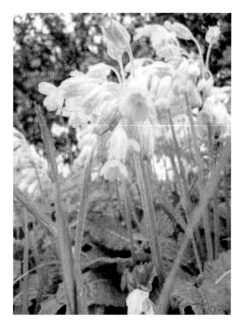

Also known as: paigles, fairy cups, keyflower, key of heaven,
mayflower, plumrocks, drelip

Family Primulaceae.

Habitat and description Cowslip has leaves that grow in
basal rosettes, much like those of the primrose. The leaves are
oval and wrinkled, with interesting curling around the edges
of the younger leaves; the flowers form on long stems that
nod up to 15 cm (6 in.) above the basal rosette and are pale
yellow, with a darker yellow-orange at the throat. Interestingly,
cowslips have two different sorts of flowers, which are not

found on the same plant. Pin flowers have a long style and short stamens, with the stigma sitting at the opening of the corolla. Thrum flowers have the stigma located deep in the corolla, with the anthers at the opening. Much beloved of bees, cowslips were, for a while, becoming increasingly rare in the wild. These days they can be found in wild ground, meadows, forest and woodland edges, gardens and verges, as council initiatives to plant wildflower verges have helped to restore the number of them growing in the UK. There are several fields near my home that are filled with cowslips every spring, which is a very beautiful sight. Cowslips will readily cross with primroses to create oxlips, which are not much used in herbal medicine though still much beloved of bees and insects.

Where to find it   Temperate Europe, including the milder parts of Scandinavia, and parts of Asia. Other parts of the world have their own native versions of the same plant family.

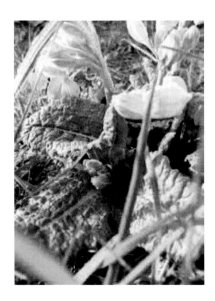

Parts used   The whole plant is used – flowers, leaves and root – gathered at different times of the year.

When to gather   The first few flowers will appear in March and can be picked from then all through the summer flowering season, but be careful not to overharvest from any one plant: leave plenty for the bees and enough to allow the plants to set seed, especially if you would like to increase your cowslip patch over the coming year. The leaves can be gathered from late March onwards – I tend to wait until April, though, as the leaves are more sturdy, more open, and less crinkly by then, and the weather is milder. Drying them in March can be slightly more tricky, as the weather is much damper and the rain and dew tends to get caught in the leaf folds. The root can be dug in the autumn, when the plant has gone dormant, but take roots only from your own garden, as they have been very scarce in the wild in the UK. Mark where the plant is in late summer if you plan to unearth the root, and dig it up for tincturing from October onwards.

Medicines to make   Cowslips can be used to make a range of medicines, including – but certainly not limited to – infused oils, balms and salves. Tinctures and elixirs provide medicines for taking over the winter, while teas and infused wines can be made using the fresh flowers and enjoyed seasonally. A particularly lovely remedy is cowslip honey, made by finely chopping the flowers and mixing into local honey. The flowers can also be eaten on their own: they taste predominantly of dried apricots, with a hint of floral flavours.

Constituents   Saponin glycosides, flavonoids, tannins, to name but a few.

Planetary influence   Venus.

Associated deities and heroes   Freya, Blodeuwedd, spring goddesses. Heavily linked with many of the faery queens as well.

Festival   Ostara.

Constitution   Cool and moist.

Actions and indications   Cowslip has long been used as a sedative and is well suited to those with anxiety and over-active brains; it is also useful for nervous headache and sleeplessness, and for restlessness in children, for which it combines well with German chamomile. For these uses it is best taken as a tea, but it also makes a very tasty elixir with brandy and honey. It can be used for panic attacks and to soothe irritability.

The flowers contain fairly high quantities of flavonoids, which are anti-inflammatory and anti-spasmodic, making it a great herb for the relief of joint discomfort. Also, due to a combination of sedative and anti-inflammatory properties, it has been used for nerve tremors, such as those caused by Parkinson's.

A decoction of the whole plant can be used for circulatory problems, including varicose veins and intermittent claudication, as well as for high blood pressure; use it with caution in the latter, however, especially if you are already being treated for this. Internally and externally it can be used to relieve rheumatism and arthritis.

It also has an affinity with the lungs, and a tea of the plant can provide relief for bronchitis, whooping cough and other chest-related issues. It does this through a stimulant–expectorant effect on the lungs, encouraging the body to remove excess phlegm. I've found other sources that consider the root to be better suited to the lungs, but try both and see which works best for you. As with many herbs, it is a case of using what is available, beginning with the more gentle remedy, then, if the flower doesn't have the desired effect, progressing to more robust treatments using the root.

Folklore   Very much the same as the primrose, covered elsewhere in this book – these two plants are heavily linked and are often used interchangeably. Folk tales link it with fairy-land: several versions of the same basic tale speak of a young girl gaining access to fairyland using cowslips or primroses, depending on the version told.

Dose   One teaspoon of flowers and leaves to a cup of hot water to make a tea, drunk twice a day; 5 ml twice a day of the tincture or elixir.

Contraindications   Large doses are emetic, probably due to the presence of saponins. The roots contain salicylates, so if you are allergic to these, avoid or use with caution. Both cowslip and primrose can cause contact dermatitis in some people, so if you are prone to this, be cautious.

Cowslip recipes

Cowslip elixir

Ingredients

» plenty of freshly picked cowslip flowers and leaves – at least 1 pint, loosely packed (try to gather these from your own garden or from other cultivated sources if possible, and ensure you go for the wild version instead of the cultivars)
» vodka or brandy
» local honey

Instructions   As with all recipes using fresh plant matter, check over your flowers and leaves carefully to make sure they are clean and free from pests, then chop up finely. Pack them into a Kilner jar – the 1-l (1¾-pint) size works well – and pour over the brandy to just cover the plant matter, adding a large tablespoon or two of local honey. Put the lid on the jar and shake it up thoroughly. Put the jar in a dark place and leave for a fortnight, shaking it up every day or every other day; at the end of that time, strain the mixture through a sieve and some kitchen roll or muslin. Bottle the resulting liquid and store in a dark cupboard. A good dose is 5 ml twice a day for sore joints, arthritis, and also for coughs and colds. It can also be used to ease you towards a restful night's sleep, truly a multipurpose remedy! An alcohol-free version of this can be made by omitting the vodka and honey and covering the plant matter with vegetable glycerine instead.

This recipe can also be made combining violets, cowslips and rose petals – just leave the elixir in a jar and add flowers as they bloom, going for roughly equal amounts of each plant.

Cowslip tincture

This recipe is an ongoing process, utilising all three parts of the plant – flowers, leaves and roots –starting in April and finishing in November. It can either be added to as the various parts of the plant are harvested, or you can make separate tinctures of each and then blend and store as a combined tincture.

Ingredients
- » 1 pint, roughly, of cowslip flowers
- » 1 pint, roughly, of cowslip leaves
- » 1 tbsp chopped (roughly) of cowslip roots
- » 500 ml (17½ fl oz) of brandy or vodka, the strongest you can get hold of

Instructions   Finely chop the leaves and flowers using a sharp knife, mezzaluna or the food processor, and pack them into a Kilner jar, then pour over the alcohol. Put the lid on and label it carefully.

In the autumn, repeat the process, using the roots instead of the leaves and flowers. Clean the roots well and chop them finely, then add them to the jar on top of the leaves and flowers.

If you would rather prepare a separate root tincture, put 4 tbsp (60 g) of roots, cleaned and chopped, into a jar and cover them with alcohol, with an extra 2.5 cm (1 in) on top; seal and label, then leave the whole lot to steep for at least two weeks – a month is often better with root remedies.

The flower and leaf tincture can ease panic attacks and anxiety and can also be used to cool down an overactive brain that is not allowing restful sleep. I suggest a 1-tsp dose of the leaves and flowers tincture.

To relieve chesty coughs and bronchitis, use 10 drops of the root tincture, taken no more than once every two to three hours.

With the tincture made from leaves, flowers and roots, or if you have combined the separate tinctures into one, then this can be used in the same way as the separate tinctures, but for a wider spectrum of symptoms, where each different plant part builds on and reinforces the properties of the others. You may find you will need lower doses if you use the tincture of the whole plant, so begin with 5 drops rather than 10, and increase gradually from there. Too much may cause nausea.

Cowslip honey

Ingredients
- » 1 pint of loosely packed, fresh cowslip flowers
- » 1 jar of local runny honey

Instructions   Using a mezzaluna or a food processor, finely chop the clean flowers and then stir them carefully into a whole jar of local runny honey. You will almost certainly need to decant the mixture into a larger jar first! Store the mixture in a dark cupboard and let it infuse for at least a month. Take one teaspoon of cowslip honey to relieve anxiety, encourage a good night's sleep and soothe irritating coughs and colds. You can also stir it into a cup of cowslip tea for the same purpose, to obtain a double hit of the same herb.

Whole cowslip decoction

Ingredients
- » 1 tbsp (15 g approx.) each of cowslip flowers and leaves
- » 1 tsp (5 g approx.) of chopped cowslip root
- » 570 ml (20 fl oz) of water

Instructions   Ideally, dig up the cowslip root very early in the spring, before the plant flowers – you will almost certainly need to sacrifice a plant for this. Scrub the roots clean, finely chop them, and freeze them in a labelled jar until you need them. When you want to make the decoction, gather the flowers and leaves from the garden and finely chop them, then add them with the frozen root to a pan of water. Pop a lid on and bring the whole lot to a steady simmer; let it simmer for at least half an hour, an hour being better if possible, until the liquid has reduced down by at least a third. Take it off the heat and strain out the herbs, then sweeten it with a little honey. Take 1-tbsp doses (10–15 ml) up to four times a day for coughs, colds and bronchitis. This will keep for up to three days in the fridge – you may find freezing the rest in ice-cube trays would be a good idea, so that you have it for future occasions.

Daisy
Bellis perennis

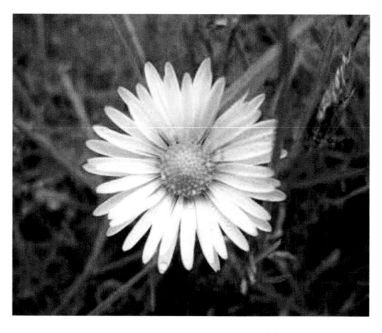

Also known as: bruisewort, bairnwort, llygad y dydd (eye of the day —
Welsh), flower of spring, gowan, open eye, day's eye, banwood, banewort,
ewe-gowan, little star, silver pennies, billy button, measure of love, herb
Margaret, bainswort, bruisewort, child's flower, field daisy, maudlinwort,
moon daisy

Family Asteraceae.

Habitat and description Daisies are commonly found in
proliferation growing in lawns and grassy verges, and they
can flower extremely thickly from early spring through until
autumn. The leaves lie in a flat basal rosette and are both
juicy and lightly hairy, with the flowers rising to a height of

perhaps 5 cm (2 in), at most, from the leaves. This shape is extremely useful, as it means that lawn mowers often pass straight over the top of them, much to the disgust of some gardeners who would prefer their lawns without the presence of flowers such as the daisy. The plant is also found in meadows and uncultivated pastures, as well as growing between flagstones. Most people could correctly identify a daisy: the many-petalled white flowers with their sunny centres are an extremely familiar sight. Sometimes on the underside of the petals the flowers have a coloured edge, ranging from pale pink to magenta, making them really stand out.

Where to find it   Europe and most of America.

Parts used   Flowers and leaves; roots.

When to gather   Flowers and leaves from May through the summer, roots in the autumn. The flowers can be picked and put to dry in hydroponic drying racks or shallow baskets, where they can be flicked into the air every other day to turn them over. The roots will need to be cleaned, chopped and dehydrated for storage.

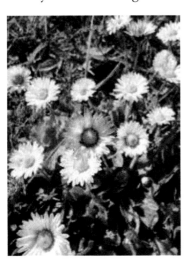

Medicines to make   Daisy-infused oil and balm for bumps, bruises and sore joints. Daisy syrup, tincture or elixir for chesty coughs and other things. Dried daisy flowers for the store cupboard.

Constituents   Bitters, mucilage and saponins. Essential oil – around 20% polyacetylenes. Tannins and flavones, as well as resins.

Planetary influence   Daisy is predominantly ruled by Venus but also has some links with the moon.

Associated deities and heroes   Freya, Artemis and Thor, Zeus, Aphrodite and Venus; Alcestis, Apollo, Belenos – quite a few of the main "father" gods from a variety of pantheons. I'd also link it with deities working with spring, fresh starts and innocence.

Festival   The Equinoxes, perhaps especially the spring equinox and the pagan festival of Ostara.

Constitution   Gently cool and dry.

Actions and indications   In his *Herball*, John Gerard was of the opinion that "the daisy do mitigate all kinds of paines, but especially in the joints, and gout ... the leaves stamped take away bruises and swellings proceeding of some stroke, if they be stamped and laid thereon; whereupon it was called in old time Bruisewort." I certainly use it for this, to good effect, as it is easy to obtain, does not cause the breakdown of skin cells, and is very effective – it combines beautifully with elder bark and leaves and yarrow leaves to make a superb all-purpose bruise and bump balm. As this balm is perfectly safe and healing to use on cuts and grazes, it can also be used for minor injuries. Culpeper used it in his time to treat ulcers of the mouth and genitalia, as well as inflammation associated with local wounds. He also stated that "the juice or distilled water . . . doth much temper the heat of choler, and refresh the liver, and other inward parts."

The main action of the plant is astringent and tonic, making it very useful for issues arising from hyper-relaxed veins and mucous membranes or broken skin. These days it is used to treat a variety of complaints, ranging from circulatory to respiratory issues, as well as the well-known uses to treat inflammation, both internally and externally. It is anti-inflammatory, a vasotonic alterative, antifungal and antibacterial, as well as being anti-viral, and a cardiac tonic. The plant is also diuretic and diaphoretic, helping to lower fevers, as well as being anti-rheumatic, antispasmodic, anodyne and vulnerary, all properties linked with pain relief and healing. These uses all seem to agree with those provided in their herbals by Gerard and Culpeper. Basically, daisy does a bit of everything, making it a really handy tonic to have in the cupboard!

The root is used as an alterative to cleanse the blood of toxins and uric acid, making it handy to relieve gout and most inflammatory diseases affecting the joints, as well as to ease skin disorders. The plant can also be used as a circulatory tonic, improving blood supply to the peripheral circulation.

Because of its expectorant properties, the daisy can also be used to treat respiratory ailments such as coughs and catarrh – though mind the dosage, as the presence of saponins can cause a bout of nausea if you take too much of the herb. As an astringent, it can be used to dry up inflammatory diseases affecting internal mucous membranes, such as gastroenteritis and bronchitis, as well as externally for a variety of skin disorders and eruptions. Around the eyes, an ointment can ease inflammation and bruising – handy for martial artists, perhaps, but hopefully most people will be fortunate enough to not require it for such purposes!

Folklore   The simple daisy has a wide and long-lasting body of folklore surrounding it. To begin with, there are several theories surrounding the Latin name of Bellis, as some authors believe it is derived from the Latin word "bellus" meaning "pretty", whereas others believe that it derives from the word "bello", which is Latin for "war": this association may be due to the plant's long-standing reputation as a wound herb, as well as the fact that it may well have been found growing on or near most battlefields. This association may perhaps partially explain the dichotomy between the assorted deities with which the plant is associated.

There is also the possibility that the name derives from the myth of the water meadow nymph, Belidis, who changed herself into a daisy in order to avoid the amorous attentions of the orchard god Vertumnus. The plant's name has also been associated with the Celtic sun god, Belenos. The name "daisy" derives from the Anglo Saxon name for the plant, "daeges eage", which means "day's eye", alluding to the plant's tendency to open only during sunlit hours.

The old authors – most notably Gerard and Culpeper – believed that the root of the daisy could be used to stunt growth, and the plant was often given to puppies to keep them small.

The folk name "Measure of Love" comes from the old tradition of plucking petals from a daisy while reciting "he loves me, he loves me not" as a simple love divination charm.

Dried daisies picked between noon and one o'clock before drying bring success to any venture, according to an old piece of German folklore.

Dose   One teaspoon of dried herb to one cup of hot water can be infused and drunk up to four times a day. The recommended tincture dosage is 2–4 ml of the tincture three times a day.

Contraindications   The herb should be used sparingly, as the presence of saponins can prove irritant to the digestion.

Daisy recipes

Daisy, elder and yarrow bruise balm

Ingredients
- » 1 pint, loosely packed, of equal amounts of fresh elder leaves and bark, daisy flowers and yarrow leaves
- » organic vegetable oil
- » beeswax
- » peppermint and rosemary essential oils

Instructions   Finely dice the herbs and put them into the top of a double boiler with the oil, making sure the herbs are thoroughly covered – allow 5 mm of extra oil on top of the herbs. Simmer gently until the oil changes colour, strain out the herbs, and allow 12 g beeswax to 100 ml (3½ fl oz) of oil. Warm and stir until the beeswax melts, then add 10 drops each of peppermint and rosemary essential oils, stir briefly, and pour into jars.

This balm is suitable for all kinds of bruises and bumps and is also safe to use on minor cuts and grazes, making it a great all-purpose balm.

Daisy and yarrow wound spray

Ingredients
- » ¼ pint, lightly pressed down, of daisy flowers and leaves
- » a roughly equal amount of yarrow leaves
- » vodka

Instructions   Finely chop all the herbs and pile them into a clean glass jar – a large jam or preserving jar works well. Pour over the vodka and put the lid on, letting the herbs steep for a fortnight, then filter out the herbs and put the resulting alcohol into pump spray bottles. Label them carefully. This spray can be used for cuts and grazes, to clean them and encourage them to heal properly.

Daisy elixir

Ingredients
- » ¼ pint of daisy leaves and flowers
- » 2 tbsp (30 g approx.) of daisy roots
- » brandy
- » local honey

Instructions   Finely chop all the ingredients and pile them into a jar; add 15 g of local honey, and then top up with enough brandy to cover the herbs and honey. Shake it up thoroughly, then pack the herbs under the level of the alcohol again. Steep the whole lot for a fortnight, then strain out the herbs. Take 10 drops in a little water for coughs and bronchitis, to help the body remove excess phlegm. You can also take 10 drops regularly to improve rheumatism and arthritis, and even as a cardiac tonic, though if you are using it for the latter purpose, do make sure you have a medical professional helping you to monitor your blood pressure.

Daisy cough syrup

Ingredients
- » ½ pint of loosely packed daisy flowers and leaves
- » 570 ml (20 fl oz) of water
- » zest and juice of one lemon
- » brown sugar

Instructions   Shred the flowers thoroughly and cover them with the water, then add the zest and juice of the lemon and bring the whole lot to a gentle simmer for half an hour, until the liquid amount has reduced by a quarter. Strain the herbs through a muslin cloth — the flowers and lemon can be composted. Return the liquid to the clean saucepan, and add 500 g (1 lb 1½ oz) of sugar. Warm the mixture, stirring it regularly until the sugar has dissolved, then bring it to a boil and simmer it for 5 minutes, until it has thickened slightly. Bottle it hot, and label it once it has cooled. Take 1 tsp (5 ml) up to three times a day for stubborn coughs where the phlegm refuses to shift.

Dandelion
Taraxacum officinale

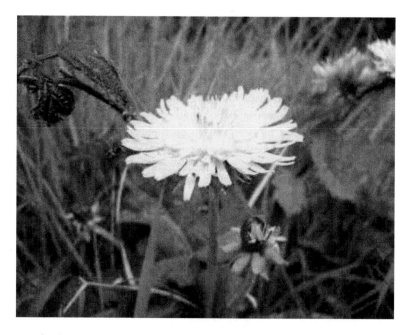

Also known as: witch gowan, devil's milk plant, lion's teeth, golden
suns, clocks and watches, piss a bed, stink davie, heart fever grass, dog
posy, blowball, peasant's clock, cankerwort, crow-parsnip, irish daisy,
doon-head-clock, fortune teller, one o'clocks, swinesnout, wet-a-bed,
shit-a-bed, bum-pie, burning fire, clocks, combs and hairpins, conquer
more, devil's milk pail, fairy clocks, farmer's clocks, horse gowan, lay-a-
bed, male, mess-a-bed, pishamoolag, pissimire, pittle bed, priest's crown,
schoolboy's clocks, shepherd's clock, stink davine, tell-time, time flower,
time teller, twelve o'clock, wishes, wet-weed, white endive, wild endive
(to name but a few!)

Family   Asteraceae.

Habitat and description   Dandelion pops up in many different places – from wasteland, scrub, roadsides, lawns and meadows to the patches in the garden that you would really rather were dandelion-free! The jagged-edged, lance-shaped leaves are plentiful, forming a basal rosette from which the flower stems rise, with tall, hairless, hollow stems topped by the bright yellow, many-petalled flower heads much loved and needed by bees as one of their first sources of food in spring. The plant blooms from March until May and often again between July and September. The rather pretty flower heads are followed by the familiar dandelion clock, or seed head, so beloved of children, and the air-borne mechanism of the plant allows it to set seed readily. The leaves can vary from small, barely 5 cm (2 in) long, to 30 cm (12 in) or longer, depending on where it is growing, and it can worm its way into the smallest of gaps with little to no soil.

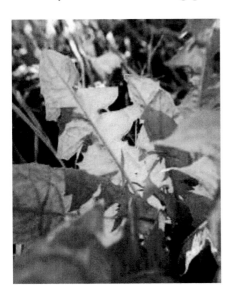

Where to find it   Pretty much every temperate zone can boast some form of dandelion, and there are indeed thousands of different cultivars to choose from, all of which are used in a similar fashion.

Parts used   The whole plant – flowers, leaves and roots – is used for different purposes.

When to gather   Flowers can be picked in April and May, and leaves can be collected from March to May. Roots can be dug either in very early spring for more bitter roots, as the plant has used its stores of nutrients to last through the winter, or late September through to November for sweeter roots, as it has had the summer to absorb and transmute sun into sugars.

Medicines to make   Tinctures can be made from the leaf or the root. Infused oil of the flowers is a lovely thing to create, to turn into salves and ointments. Elixirs of the root are beneficial to the digestive system. The sap from the stem is useful in the treatment of warts, although it should not be taken internally, as it is slightly toxic, especially to children.

Constituents   Sesquiterpene lactones, taraxacoside, taraxinic acid, dihydrotaraxinic acid and taraxacolide glucosides, etc., as well as polyphenolic caffeoyltartaric acids, coumarins, triterpenes such as taraxol, taraxerol and taraxasterol, beta amyrin, stimgasterol and beta sitosterol. It has a higher vitamin A content than carrots. It also contains potassium, bitter glycoside, triterpenoids, tannins and mucilage.

Planetary influence   Jupiter.

Associated deities and heroes   Hecate, St George, Theseus.

Festival   Beltane, Samhain.

Constitution   Warm and moist.

Actions and indications   Dandelion enjoys a long history of use in herbal medicine, for the treatment of a wide array of ailments.

The root of the plant contains most of the bitter principles that have an action on the liver, and it can be used to build up liver tissue, making it useful in the treatment of cirrhosis, hepatitis, jaundice, gall stones and chronic liver congestion. It is also useful in treating ailments of the circulatory system, such as varicose veins and haemorrhoids, and is a blood cleanser, making it of benefit in the treatment of rheumatism, gout, and chronic skin conditions. It is a non-irritant remedy for constipation and can be used to remove toxins from the system (remember the old dandelion-and-burdock drink?). It can also be used for chronic, deep-seated illnesses such as glandular fever as a strengthening tonic. The presence of inulin and its action on the liver and pancreas mean that dandelion can be used to improve blood sugar management in the body, making it very well suited for metabolic syndrome, the precursor to diabetes.

The leaf is a useful diuretic, with a high potassium level, making it very suitable for any kind of water retention, especially where this is due to cardiac failure. It is demulcent and healing to the kidneys and bladder and can be used to treat cystitis and other inflammations of the urinary tract. It can also be used to treat lung complaints such as bronchitis and asthma, as it strengthens the lung tissue.

Dandelion root has a strong affinity for most of the digestive system, including the pancreas and gallbladder. The bitters in it stimulate the appetite and regulate digestion. It is a mild laxative and choleretic and contains vitamins A, B and C, as well as being rich in minerals. It is used to treat inflammation of the gall bladder and to relieve jaundice, and for indigestion, anorexia, cachexia and related wasting disease. The milky sap from the stem is applied fresh to warts.

I have used dandelion root alongside other herbs in the relief of mild to moderate depression, especially where this is caused by stuck "fire" in the liver. Take a look at the tongue – if it is red, with lots of fine lines and cracks, a central fissure and some coating, then this is a pretty good indication that dandelion root will be useful. I've also used it to regulate the liver, which, in turn, will affect hormone levels due to increased levels of excretion of spent or excess hormones.

Folklore The wide variety of charming – and not so charming – names for dandelion portray many of the folkloric beliefs associated with it as well as reflecting its properties as a strong diuretic. The dandelion seed heads, or clocks, have a plentiful array of folk practices associated with them. If you whisper thoughts about a loved one to the seed head, then blow the seeds off, the wind will carry your words along with the seeds to the loved one in question. In addition to this, several different versions of folklore are associated with the number of seeds left on the seed head after one good, hard puff – ranging from how many years before they will marry, how many children they will bear or father, to the number of years a person has left to live.

Dose Up to 4 tsp of leaf per cup of tea, or 1 tsp of root to one cup of boiling water decocted for 15 minutes – the dosage of both tea and decoction being ½–1 cup, taken freely. The dosage for the liquid extract is up to 2 tsp, and that for the tincture is up to 10 ml of 1:5 25% per day.

Contraindications Excessive doses can cause slight nausea and diarrhoea; dandelion should be avoided in cases of excess stomach heat such as acid indigestion, as it can worsen it.

Dandelion recipes

Dandelion petal butter

Ingredients / equipment
- » one handful of fresh dandelion flowers
- » honey
- » one large pot of double cream
- » one large empty Kilner jar with watertight lid

Instructions   This recipe is great fun to make but quite hard work, so definitely worth sharing with friends or family if possible! I suggest doing this in two equal parts, to make it a little quicker. First, make sure your cream is warm – room temperature at least, but slightly warmer than that is even better. If it is fresh out of the fridge, put it on a sunny windowsill for an hour, or stand it in a basin of warm water for a while, shaking it up regularly to mix the cooler cream with the freshly warmed stuff. Then pour half the pot into the jar, put the lid on, and begin shaking it. Keep shaking it regularly for at least 20 minutes, by which time you should start to notice some solids in the jar – this is the beginning of the butter forming. Keep shaking until your arms start to get really tired, or until you see substantial amounts of butter solids, whichever comes first! Pour the resulting mixture through a sieve into a jug. The liquid left is the buttermilk, which can be used in a nettle soup recipe or instead of regular milk while making pancakes. The solids is basically now butter! Now comes the fun bit.

Using two forks and a plate, mash the butter solids thoroughly, tipping regularly to pour off any other buttermilk trapped between the small lumps of butter. Keep doing this until most of the buttermilk has gone.

For this sweet butter, remove all the green bits from the

dandelion petals and roughly chop the petals, then mash into the butter. Sweeten with either honey or brown sugar – I tend to prefer brown sugar, as it keeps a good texture that way. Runny honey can sometimes dilute it a bit too much – set honey works better. This sweetened butter can be spread onto bread or crackers as a delicious sweet treat!

(*See also* Jack-by-the-hedge butter.)

Dandelion flower spelt bread

Ingredients
- » 500 g (1 lb 1½ oz) spelt flour
- » 300 ml (10 fl oz) water
- » ½ pint of dandelion flowers
- » 1 dessertspoon of dried yeast
- » a pinch of salt
- » 2 dessertspoons of brown sugar for the bread, and 1 tsp to start the yeast rising

Instructions First, mix 50 ml (1¾ fl oz) boiling water with 1 tsp of brown sugar until the sugar has mostly dissolved. Add 100 ml (3½ fl oz) of cold water and stir in thoroughly, then add the yeast and whisk in. Put the jug onto a warm, sunny windowsill for 10 minutes to allow the yeast to start rising. Meanwhile, weigh out the spelt flour and add the yellow dandelion petals, minus the green bits, plus the salt and the 2 dessertspoonfuls of brown sugar. Mix it thoroughly. Make a well in the middle and, whisking up the yeast mixture, pour it in, then measure another 150 ml (5¼ fl oz) of water (or the buttermilk left over from the recipe above) swishing it around in the jug to pick up all the remaining yeast. Pour that in as well. Using a wooden spoon, work the mixture into a rough batter. Then it's time to get your hands dirty! Thoroughly dusting a table top with a handful of the flour, give the dough a good kneading until the gluten strands start to stretch and the consistency changes a little. The dough should begin to feel more elastic and almost alive in your hands. Form it into small balls, and put these onto a tray to rise for 45 minutes before you put them into the oven. Heat the oven to 170°C, and put the bread rolls in for 20 minutes, keeping an eye on them. Spelt sometimes has the entertaining habit of trying to escape the oven! The bread rolls are done when they sound hollow when you tap them on the bottom with a knuckle. Leave them to cool slightly, covering with a tea towel if you prefer soft crusts, and enjoy them with dandelion or Jack-by-the-hedge herb butter and a bowl of savoury nettle soup.

Dandelion flower balm for sore muscles

Ingredients
- » 1 pint, loosely packed, of dandelion flowers
- » organic rapeseed oil
- » beeswax pellets
- » cedar essential oil

Instructions   Chop the dandelion flowers roughly, and put them into the top of the double boiler, pouring over the rapeseed oil and simmering gently for at least 30 minutes for the beneficial properties to leach out into the liquid. Strain out the dandelion flowers, and put the oil back into the double boiler with 12 g of beeswax to each 100 ml ($3\frac{1}{2}$ fl oz) of oil. Warm and stir gently until the beeswax has dissolved, then add 10 drops of cedarwood oil per 100 ml ($3\frac{1}{2}$ fl oz) of your oil. Stir briefly and pour the balm into clean, dry jars.

Apply this balm to sore joints and muscles, and to muscles sore due to stress-related issues.

Dandelion digestive bitters

Ingredients
- » vodka or brandy
- » fresh dandelion root (spring dug if possible for higher levels of bitters)
- » fresh dandelion leaves
- » filter coffee
- » orange zest or peel
- » lemon zest or peel

Instructions   Bitters are really very simple to make and can be stored in a dropper bottle, so that you can take a few drops half an hour before meals. Dig up at least one large, fresh dandelion root, before flowering if possible, and scrub it thoroughly, keeping the leaves to one side. Chop the root up finely and use a mortar and pestle to bash it – you want to really bruise and open the surface and increase the surface area to allow the alcohol to get to the roots. Pile the chopped roots into a jar, and add the chopped leaves. Add 1 tsp, heaped, of good-quality filter coffee and 1 tbsp, heaped, each, of the orange and lemon zest, then pour over enough brandy to cover the herbs and peels. Put the lid on and shake it up thoroughly, then leave it to infuse for a good fortnight. Decant the liquid and pour it into a dropper bottle. Take several drops half an hour before meals to really stimulate the flow of digestive enzymes, in order to improve appetite and digestion.

Dandelion root tincture

Ingredients
- » plenty of fresh dandelion root
- » brandy or vodka

Instructions   Scrub the freshly unearthed dandelion roots thoroughly and chop up finely, then either pop into a dehydrator for an hour or so, or put into a low oven with the door ajar. This will help some of the water content to evaporate off, making a stronger tincture overall. Once the roots have dried down by about 50%, pile them into a jar and pour over the vodka or brandy, then put the lid on, shake up thoroughly, and leave for at least a fortnight. Decant the liquid and bottle it. This will be a rather bitter dandelion root tincture that will be well suited to stimulating and supporting the digestive system. The autumn root tincture is sweeter and better suited to the liver as a tonic herb, though for the best possible benefits, make equal amounts in both April and October, then mix the two together.

A good dose is 5 ml in the morning, or 2.5 ml in the morning and the same in the afternoon, to support healthy digestion. A version of this can be made using dandelion leaves, which act as a diuretic, removing excess water from the system, as well as having some bladder and kidney antiseptic properties, though kidney and bladder remedies are often better taken as a tea.

Dandelion and liquorice elixir

Ingredients
- » fresh dandelion root, unearthed either in the spring or the autumn
- » dried or fresh liquorice root
- » cinnamon powder
- » brandy

Instructions   Wash and finely chop the dandelion roots, either putting them into a blender or grating them. Put at least 3 tbsp, heaped, of the grated root into a Kilner jar, along with an equivalent amount of liquorice root, dried or fresh, and at least 1 tsp, heaped, of cinnamon, then pour over plenty of brandy. I tend to suggest covering by two finger widths for this one as the water content in the dandelion root will slightly water down the brandy. You shouldn't need to add honey, as the liquorice will sweeten it up thoroughly anyway.

Take 5 ml of the elixir three times a day in a case of polycystic ovary syndrome (PCOS) and for liver-related issues, including metabolic syndrome – the precursor to diabetes. Do not, however, use this elixir if you are taking metformin or other diabetes medications, unless you are having the process closely monitored to ensure blood sugar remains stable.

Greater celandine
Chelidonium majus

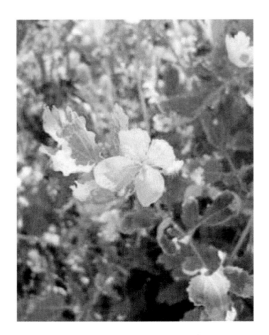

Also known as: common celandine, garden celandine, swallow herb, wartweed

Family   Papaveraceae.

Habitat and description   This beautiful, short-lived perennial springs back to life early each year, producing clumps of attractive, frilly, deeply divided bright-green foliage and bright-yellow four-petalled flowers in clusters. In time, these give way to long green seed pods with black seeds in them, much beloved of birds – which might explain greater celandine's tendency to pop up in some rather odd places. The plant's stem is robust and, when broken, gives a bright orange sap that stains the skin and has a strong and rather acrid scent to it. Greater celandine is one of the earlier of the flowering spring and summer plants and will often continue to flower through to early autumn before it goes dormant. The leaves gather dew and raindrops easily, which they display in silvery, crystalline profusion. It is rather a beautiful plant, and certainly a welcome sight in the spring, a useful member of the wild garden in particular.

Greater celandine grows happily in waste ground, hedgerows and verges, tucked into the garden and anywhere else it can sneak in.

Where to find it   Europe, UK, Mediterranean countries, parts of Asia and North America, where it has naturalized.

Parts used   The whole fresh plant, gathered while in flower and dried in bunches, or tinctured fresh.

When to gather   May and June.

Medicines to make   A weak cottage tincture of the fresh plant can be made; the juice can be useful for warts and corns.

Constituents   Alkaloids, including chelidonine and homochelidonine A and B; protopine, sanguinarine and bitter principles; flavonoids; fruit acids; proteolytic enzymes.

Planetary influence   Sun.

Associated deities and heroes   Any deities linked with the sun – no surprise, given the glorious colour of the flowers.

Festival   Beltane and Ostara.

Constitution   Hot and dry.

Actions and indications   Greater celandine isn't quite so widely used as a remedy these days, but in the past it enjoyed quite a reputation for a variety of different ailments. These days it is predominantly used as a liver and pancreatic herb, boosting and improving the health of these organs; it is used to treat jaundice and bile imbalances. In addition to this, it is a useful remedy for inefficient liver function resulting in headaches, and also for migraines with light sensitivity. Celandine can be used to decongest the pancreas.

Celandine also possesses some antispasmodic properties, which, linked with the liver and gallbladder, make it very useful for pain and congestion in these organs. Recently it has also been used for asthma, as it has an affinity for the lungs. As a result of this, it can also be used as part of a remedy for spasmodic coughs, and as it has an affinity with the central nervous system, it can also be part of remedies where there is tension in this area.

Fresh celandine juice can be applied carefully to warts, ringworm and corns, making sure you don't get any on the surrounding skin.

Ointments, balms and salves can be made from the roots for piles and varicose veins.

In Russia, the whole plant has a history as a cancer remedy and, indeed, at least one of the constituents has been shown to slow down cell division in cancer cells. It has been used to break down uterine fibroids and even abdominal tumours.

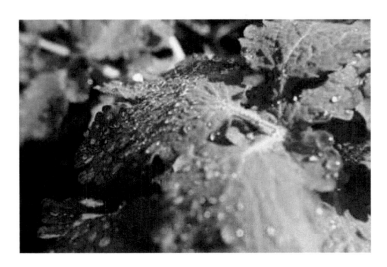

The plant has a long history of use for the eyes, particularly for glaucoma, cataracts and conjunctivitis.

Folklore   Pliny named it "chelidonium", after the swallows, as it flowers when the swallows first arrive and fades when the swallows leave again.

Amulets of celandine are said to soothe quarrelsome personalities, calming aggressive people.

Dose   Of the weak tincture, 1:6 25%, single-drop doses.

Contraindications   Use very cautiously, as this remedy is very strong indeed.

Greater celandine recipes

Celandine juice for warts

Ingredients
» 1 freshly cut small stem of celandine

Instructions   Cut the stem using sharp scissors and let the sap run until it begins to turn orange, then turn it so the cut side is upside down, and apply it carefully to the wart. Try not to let the juice touch the rest of the skin, just the wart itself. Let the sap dry. Repeat this process once or twice a day, until the wart has gone.

Celandine and dandelion root cottage tincture for liver health

Ingredients
» 1 pint, loosely packed, of dandelion root
» ½ pint, loosely packed, of celandine tops, including the flowers
» brandy or vodka

Instructions   Scrub clean the dandelion roots, preferably gathered before the plant has flowered, then finely chop them and put them into a Kilner jar, covering them with enough of the chosen alcohol to allow an extra 2.5 cm (1 in) on top of the roots. These may need to be left to infuse for a few weeks while the celandine wakes up and puts on some spring growth – no need to worry if this is the case, just give the jar a shake regularly to turn the roots over. Once the celandine has sprouted, pick some of the tops, including the flowers. Some people have a sensitivity to the plant and its sap – so if you have allergies or intolerances to any other flowers or plants, best use gloves for this part. Check over the freshly gathered plant and then finely chop it before packing it into the Kilner jar with the dandelion root and stirring it up thoroughly to make sure the fresh leaves are well covered by the alcohol. Let the whole lot steep and infuse for a fortnight, shaking it up regularly, then strain it through kitchen paper or muslin and pop the resulting tincture into a bottle. Decant a small amount of it into a dropper bottle and take 5 drops in a little water twice a day to boost and improve digestive health.

Ground elder
Aegopodium podagraria

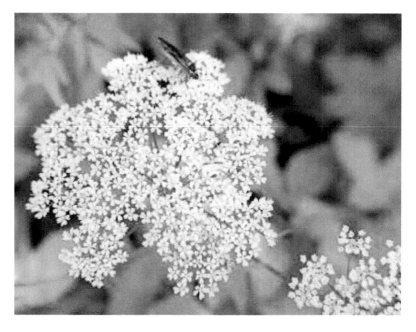

Also known as: goutweed, gout herb, ground ash, herb Gerarde, ashweed, bishopweed, bishop's wort, snow-in-the-mountain, english masterwort, Johny jump around

Family   Apiaceae.

Habitat and description   Ground elder is a much maligned denizen of many a garden, where it rambles freely wherever it fancies, tossing up shoots of leaves that bear a strong resemblance to those of the elder tree, for which it is named. It is a real nuisance to get rid of once you have it, as only the tiniest part of the root is needed for the plant to begin to merrily grow again! The first leaves appear in April – tender green things with soft stems, which can be eaten – indeed, this is the main reason the plant can be found in this country, as the Romans originally brought it here as a food crop, and the Victorians brought it over again as a ground cover, ornamental and food plant. The young leaves and shoots can be steamed and eaten like spinach, having a flavour somewhat like that of asparagus – certainly a good way of at least reducing the nuisance of having the plant in the garden. You can also add it to soups and stews or make it into pesto. Ground elder is a creeping perennial, spreading by way of fine roots. It has white or sometimes palest pink, rather feathery flowers in umbels, and the whole plant is quite strongly fragrant – a sort of cross between celery and crushed elder leaves.

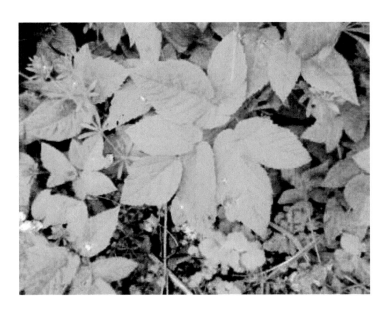

Where to find it   Most of the UK, as well as Europe, Russia, the USA, Ireland, and even as far afield as New Zealand.

Parts used   Young leaves and shoots.

When to gather   March, April and May.

Medicines to make   Tincture; dried herb for tea, salads, soups; and pesto made using the young, fresh leaves and stems.

Constituents   The main constituents are flavonoids, furanocoumarins, polyynes, volatile oils, and caffeic acid derivatives. It also contains lots of trace minerals and vitamin C, making it a useful addition to the diet.

Planetary influence   Saturn according to Culpeper.

Associated deities and heroes   I suspect a possible link with some of the same deities as elder (*Sambucus nigra*): Hel, Hela, Holda, Hilde, dryads, Earth Goddesses with a distinct link to the Underworld, fairies, crone aspects of the Goddess such as Cailleach, Hecate, Cerridwen, The Morrigan, Lilith, Kali, etc.

Festival   Beltane.

Constitution   Cool and moist.

Actions and indications   As one of the folk names suggests, goutweed was originally much used for the treatment of gout; it can often be found near monastic ruins, as it was used extensively by the well-fed bishops who often suffered from this complaint. The leaf can be used as a diuretic to reduce water retention and also has an old reputation as a sedative. Culpeper reckoned that all you needed to do was carry it with you to ward off gout!

It was extensively used in the past as a diuretic, removing wastes from the joints that cause pain linked to gout, arthritis and rheumatism. As a sedative, it can provide gentle pain relief from these conditions.

It has also been used to treat eczema when drunk as a tea on a daily basis combined with fresh dandelion leaves. The leaf and root, mashed up together, can be used as a poultice for sciatica, though it is not of benefit in all cases – I suspect it is particularly well suited to sufferers prone to excessive amounts of heat.

Hildegard of Bingen used it to treat stomach pain – so quite possibly it shares the carminative effects of so many of the Apiaceae family when drunk or eaten as a vegetable. Mrs Grieve quotes both Culpeper and Parkinson, saying that it can be used to ease high colour in people who are prone to excessive amounts of redness, so I would personally use it to moderate heat and encourage heat to circulate more properly around the body. It is not used much in modern herbal medicine – at least, not in the UK – but I think it is a source of unexplored medicine that could well be studied more (at the very least to reduce the huge patches of it that currently take over so many gardens)! I've heard some reports of it being rather laxative when eaten in larger amounts or later on in the summer, though by late summer it is usually quite coarse, certainly not much good for eating.

I have used it to great effect in the treatment of gout, combined with wild celery seed (*Apium graveolens*) and cleavers (*Galium aparine*).

Folklore   As previously mentioned, it is often found growing near monastic ruins, as it was commonly given to the bishops who often suffered from gout.

Dose   A tea made from 4–5 leaves, taken once a day. On the tincture, little information is available, but I would advise starting with 1 ml and working up from there gradually.

Contraindications   Given the presence of coumarin-derived phytochemicals, do not take this herb alongside warfarin or other blood thinners.

Ground elder recipes

Ground elder, cleavers, dandelion leaf and ground ivy detox tea

Ingredients
- » 1 tsp, heaped, of cleavers
- » 1 tsp, heaped, of ground ivy leaves and stems
- » 1 tsp, heaped, of dandelion leaf
- » 1 tsp, heaped, ground elder leaves and stems
- » 570 ml (20 fl oz) of water
- » several slices of lemon
- » honey or maple syrup, as preferred

Instructions   This tea is very simple to make: just finely chop the fresh herbs and pop them into a jug with several slices of lemon. Pour over 570 ml (20 fl oz) of boiling water and steep for 5 minutes, then strain out the herbs and sweeten as preferred.

This tea is a gentle bitter, a liver tonic and a diuretic, great for reducing water retention and kick-starting the body as the days begin to lengthen!

Ground elder pesto

Ingredients
- » plenty of the youngest, fresh ground elder shoots
- » olive oil
- » 50 g (2 oz) sunflower seeds
- » 1 clove of garlic
- » salt and pepper to taste
- » a drizzle of honey or maple syrup

Instructions   Check over the ground elder to make sure it is free from dirt or marks, then pile it into a food processor with plenty of olive oil: start with 50 ml (1¾ fl oz), and add more as the herbs are blended down. Blitz the herbs and oil into a thick green paste, adding more oil as needed, then add in 50 g (2 oz) of sunflower seeds and the roughly chopped clove of garlic. Continue to blend the mixture until it forms a chunky paste, then season to taste with salt and pepper, blend again, and add a last drizzle of honey or maple syrup. Give it one last quick blend to mix all the ingredients together, taste, and adjust the seasoning, as needed. This pesto is delicious smeared on fresh bread or on fish or vegetable kebabs, or spooned into a slice of squash and slow-roasted in the oven. It will keep for several weeks in the fridge, and can also be frozen, to preserve it for longer.

Ground elder honegar for gout

Ingredients
- » plenty of freshly picked young shoots of ground elder
- » 5 stems of young cleavers, each up to 25 cm (10 in) in length
- » unpasteurized cider vinegar
- » local honey

Instructions   Ensure that the young leaves are clean and free from any markings or blemishes, then finely chop them and the cleavers. Pile the herbs into a Kilner jar and pour over the vinegar, making sure that you allow an extra 2.5 cm (1 in) of liquid on top of the herbs. Add 2 tbsp (30 g), approximately, of honey – or, if you prefer, maple syrup. Seal the lid and store in a dark, cool place, shaking it up regularly to make sure the liquid circulates around the herbs and extracts plenty of the nutrients. Strain out the herbs and bottle the resulting honegar, tasting a little and adding more honey (or maple syrup) if you prefer it sweeter. Take 10 ml twice a day, along with dietary and lifestyle changes, to relieve gout and reduce the likelihood of recurrence. This method can be used with alcohol, but given that alcohol is often one of the main triggers and worsening factors of gout, it may be worth avoiding any and all alcohol for a time.

Ground ivy
Glechoma hederacea

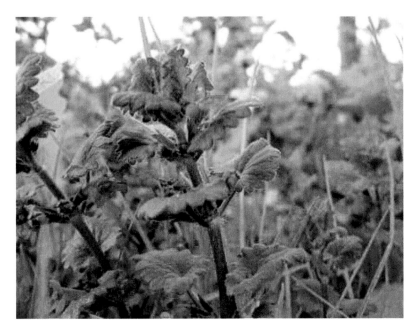

Also known as: cat's foot, gill-go-by-ground, gill-creep-by-ground, turnhoof, alehoof, haymaids, tun hoof, gill ale, gill, gill hen, hedge maids, jenny run-ith ground, jill, hayfole, heihow, heyhove, devil's candlestick, creeping charlie, lizzy-run-up-the-hedge, robin-run-up-the-hedge, field balm

Family Lamiaceae. Synonyms for *Glechoma hederacea* are *Nepeta glechoma* and *Nepeta hederacea*.

Habitat and description Ground ivy is a low-growing, creeping plant that does not usually grow to more than 20 cm (8 in) tall and so can get rather lost in the surrounding grasses. Like most other members of the mint family, it has erect, square stems and round, blunt-toothed leaves in opposing pairs. The flowers are blue-violet in colour, with three lower petals and two upper, and often with darker blue or mauve blotches. The leaves sometimes become red-tinged if the plant grows in full sun. The plant flowers between April and July, forming beautiful swathes of purple in the grasses, with a delightful aromatic fragrance when the plant is trodden upon or gathered. The bees adore it, and it is a welcome sight in spring, when the first small flowers appear in nooks and crannies.

The plant can often be found growing in woodlands, patches of scrub, and at the sides of paths, as well as in meadows and near rivers, as it likes damp soil, though I have also found it growing in plentiful array along the edges of fields in chalky ground, where it likes plenty of sun.

Where to find it   Most of Europe is home to ground ivy, as is North America.

Parts used   Leaves and flowering tops.

When to gather   April to June.

Medicines to make   Elixir made with brandy and honey; dried herb as a tea or bath or skin wash; infused wine. Combine it with plantain and nettle to relieve hayfever.

Constituents   Ground ivy contains essential oils, such as limonene and menthone, flavonoids, triterpenes such as alpha and beta ursolic acids and oleanolic acid, marrubiin, which is a diterpene, and polyphenolic acids such as rosmarinic acid. It also contains vitamin C, which perhaps accounts for its long use as a spring tonic.

Planetary influence   Venus.

Associated deities and heroes   Spring Goddesses and possibly, by extension, mythic archetypes such as Blodeuedd and other Maiden Goddesses such as Kore / Persephone.

Festival   Ostara (Spring Equinox).

Constitution   Temperate and dry.

Actions and indications   This herb has quite a wide range of therapeutic actions and uses, benefiting many different areas of the body, making it a really useful all-round remedy and a worthy member of the medicine cupboard.

Ground ivy can be used in the treatment of bladder infections, acting as a gentle diuretic and healing and toning the organ, as well as to treat cystitis and renal inflammation and kidney disease. As a dissolvant diuretic, it can be used to relieve urinary sand and stones, and the astringent properties can relieve haematuria, or blood in the urine.

It also has a wide variety of uses for the respiratory tract: to treat coughs, sinusitis, nasopharyngeal catarrh, asthma, bronchitis, nervous coughs, pertussis and tuberculosis, as well as catarrhal deafness and tinnitus. Combined with plantain, it can be used to treat sinusitis and glue ear. I also combine it regularly with plantain and nettle for hayfever.

Ground ivy can be used to treat a variety of digestive issues, including gastritis and acid indigestion, as well as diarrhoea;

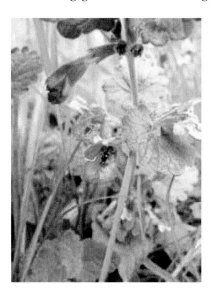

and to dry up mucous secretions. Combine it with agrimony (*Agrimonia eupatoria*) and chamomile (*Matricaria recutita*) to treat irritable bowel syndrome (IBS). It can also be used alongside other digestive herbs to treat dyspepsia, gastrointestinal ulcers, obstructive jaundice and haemorrhoids.

Topically, the herb can be used to treat nose and ear infections, and as a lotion or wash to treat lice, abscesses, itchy skin and eczema. The infused oil can be used to treat ear infections – why not combine it with mullein flower oil for this?

The herb also has a reputation as a useful nervine, particularly in the treatment of tension headaches.

Folklore   There isn't a great deal of folklore surrounding this plant; however, what is known is that the plant was widely used by the Saxons instead of hops in the production of ale, hence the name alehoof. Mrs Grieve, creator of the famous herbal encyclopaedia, was of the opinion that this was because it improved the flavour and keeping qualities of the beer and also because it made the final drink clearer.

It also has a long reputation as an excellent tisane herb, where a tea is made from the herb and is then sweetened with honey, sugar or liquorice root and allowed to cool; it is then drunk in wineglass doses, three or four times a day. In Elizabethan England it was often sold in the streets under the name "gill tea", and it was drunk as a blood purifier. Another form of this recipe was an extremely bitter version made by boiling up ground ivy and nettle tops and drinking it for nine consecutive days in the spring. This remedy was used to clear up skin complaints and as a form of spring tonic.

Dose   Standard dosage for ground ivy is tea made from 2–4 g dried herb or equivalent liquid extract three times per day. Up to 5 ml three times a day as a tincture.

Contraindications   Do not use for excessively dry conditions, as this herb will dry you out still further.

Ground ivy recipes

Ground ivy elixir

Ingredients
- » 1 pint of loosely packed ground ivy tops
- » brandy
- » honey

Instructions   Chop the clean herbs into small pieces – again, remember that the larger the surface area – that, is, the finer you chop the herbs – the more will extract into the brandy. Pack the herbs into a Kilner jar and add at least 1 tbsp (15 g) of local honey, then pour over the brandy until it covers the herbs and allows one extra 2.5 cm (1 in) of alcohol on top of the plant matter. Shake it up thoroughly, pack the herbs down again, and leave the whole lot to steep for a fortnight before straining off.

This elixir can be taken twice a day during hayfever season. To really amplify the effects, why not make the elixir using half ground ivy and half plantain? Use the elixir on its own as a super digestive and lung tonic, to strengthen the body after illness.

Ground ivy and mullein flower infused oil for the ears

Ingredients
- » plenty of young flowering ground ivy tops
- » later, mullein flowers
- » seed oil

Instructions   This infused oil very simple to make. Gather plenty of the young flowering tops on a dry day in late April, May or early June, and chop them finely before packing them into a clean jar, submerging them in seed oil, and covering the top of the jar with a piece of kitchen towel or a muslin cloth. Put the covered jar on a warm, sunny windowsill and leave it to infuse for at least two weeks, or longer – if you have a sunny, hot greenhouse, this oil can be infused there, for a quicker finish. Once you are happy with the strength of the oil, filter it through kitchen roll, bottle it and label it.

Repeat the process later in the year with mullein flowers, which you can gather on a day-by-day basis and keep adding to another jar, topping them up with the oil. Once the mullein flower oil has turned a rich yellow colour, strain out the herbs and bottle that as well. Store mullein and ground ivy oils in separate bottles, to use separately, if preferred, and also decant enough of each to fill a separate bottle, labelled to show that it contains both kinds of infused oil. You can massage it around the ear in the case of ear infections, moisten a small ball of cotton wool with it to plug the ear with, and even put a couple of drops into the ear, as long as you don't have a perforated ear drum.

Ground ivy, plantain and nettle tonic for the respiratory system

Ingredients
  - » ½ pint each, at least, of fresh ground ivy, plantain leaves and nettle tops
  - » brandy or vodka

Instructions   Check over the herbs to make sure they are clean. To make this a quicker process, I recommend checking each top as you pick it, to make sure you only take clean specimens home with you. Using a food processor or mezzaluna, finely chop the herbs, and pack them into a Kilner jar, then cover them with plenty of alcohol allowing an extra

2.5 cm (1 in) on top. Leave it to steep for at least two weeks, then strain it through muslin and bottle it. Take 1 tsp (5 ml) three times a day to strengthen the lungs, ward off hayfever, and speed up recovery from coughs and colds. If you already suffer from sinusitis or are getting over a cough, cold or chest infection, you might want to increase the dose to 10 ml up to four times a day for up to a week.

Ground ivy and mixed herb digestive tonic

Ingredients
   » plentiful amounts of any of the following herbs: ground ivy, angelica leaves, dandelion root, agrimony, sweet cicely or chamomile
   » alcohol: either brandy or vodka, depending on your preference
   » honey or maple syrup

Instructions   As with the recipe for ground ivy, plantain and nettle tonic, finely chop all the herbs and pack them into a jar, then cover them with the alcohol, allowing an extra 2.5 cm (1 in) on top. I recommend steeping the whole lot for two weeks and then trying a tiny bit of it before adding any sweetening – if you have included sweet cicely, you may find it already sweet enough for your taste without any further doctoring. Once you are happy with the blend, strain and bottle it, making a note of the ingredients, the date of bottling and the dosage – 1 tsp or 5 ml up to four times a day, to improve digestion and reduce wind, bloating and digestive disturbances.

Herb robert
Geranium robertianum

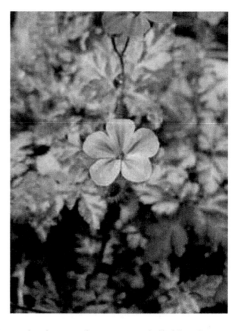

Also known as: Saint Robert's herb, St Robert, cranesbill, bloodwort, felonwort, red robin, stinking robert, death-come-quickly, cuckoo's eye, fox geranium, dragon's blood, storkbill, herb robertianum, stinky bob

Family Geraniaceae.

Habitat and description Herb robert features a fairly classic geranium family indicator in the deeply cut leaves, which grow on stems that form a basal rosette when young. The central stems are, more often than not, deep red in colour, especially in the younger plants, and the leaves themselves become deeply red later in the summer, particularly in places where they get plenty of sunlight and are on very well drained soil. Our ancestors used the particularly red plants for cuts and wounds, believing that the red colour was a clear indication of its use as a wound herb.

The plant itself becomes more leggy as it grows, sprawling in almost ferny profusion across the flower beds and borders, and features lovely, very plentiful mauve flowers from April throughout the summer, which are then followed by seeds. It self-sows quite readily and is strongly scented, a fragrance that is either loved or hated. I'm rather fond of it myself – it smells medicinal. In my garden, herb robert is always greeted with great joy every spring, wherever it has chosen to pop up.

Where to find it   Europe, Asia and North America; parts of North Africa.

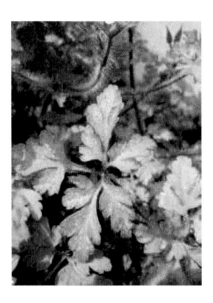

Parts used   Aerial parts – flowers, leaves and stems. The redder leaves and stems are best for topical treatments.

When to gather   May through til June or even July if the weather has been good enough.

Medicines to make   Herb-robert-infused oil, salve, ointment, plaister or cream. Herb robert tincture or elixir. Dried herb robert for teas and decoctions. Hand and foot baths.

Constituents   Germanium, apparently responsible for anti-cancer effects; flavonoids, including rutin; minerals including calcium, iron, magnesium, phosphorus and potassium; tannins; vitamins, including A, B and C; volatile oils.

Planetary influence   Venus.

Associated deities and heroes   Robin Goodfellow, Puck, Pan, Faery folk in general.

Festival   Beltane.

Constitution   Warm and temperate.

Actions and indications   Herb robert has been used internally for improving the immune system and also to treat cancer – apparently it promotes oxygen availability to cells (germanium is the main constituent that does this), which reduces the number of environments suitable for cancer to flourish in. It is especially associated with cancer that causes tumours and nodules, and it can be used both internally and externally for these sorts of issues. It makes a very good prophylactic to ward off skin cancer in susceptible people.

As an energy giver, the plant also has a reputation as an adaptogen, boosting the immune system and promoting its healthy functioning, acting as a therapeutic tonic for the whole body and as an all-round preventative of ill health.

It is a gentle bladder and kidney tonic, as the astringent and anti-inflammatory properties tighten and tone, restoring better function when the body is prone to repeat bladder and kidney infections.

It can be used to reduce swelling and improve the overall function of the liver and gallbladder, and it works to prevent stones in gallbladder, kidneys and bladder. It can be taken to relieve simple diarrhoea, especially when this is due to functional lack of tone. I have used it combined with ground ivy in alternating diarrhoea and constipation due to lack of mucous membrane and muscle tone of the bowels. It has been used in the past, alongside dietary measures, to regulate blood sugar, making it an ideal tonic for those with metabolic syndrome (the precursor to diabetes) or for those with a family history of diabetes.

It is well suited to the musculoskeletal system as well, and can be used to relieve arthritis and rheumatism and to improve circulation.

Traditionally, herb robert was used for blood problems: the colour of the stem seems to be an indicator for old, stagnant blood, varicose veins or vein congestion. It does certainly seem to make it useful for cuts, grazes and wounds, as, for this purpose, the redder the leaves and stems, the better! Herbs that have to work harder for their existence tend to show the red colouring more.

In the past, it also used to be taken to increase lactation – though without further evidence I am not sure I put a great deal of store by this, as it is astringent and could easily work the opposite way, drying up breast milk production.

Herb robert can be taken internally to encourage boils, lumps and abscesses to come to a head, drain and then heal cleanly. I would also apply it externally for this purpose.

It can be used for wounds, herpes and skin eruptions, and as a poultice for abscesses and to treat shingles, sun spots and sunburn.

It also makes a great all-round balm for bruises, cuts and grazes, for which it can be combined with plantain, also available at this time of the year.

As a poultice, it can encourage boils and abscesses to come to a head, then promote healing. You could apply a layer of the salve or ointment to a piece of cloth, pop this on the area and bandage it lightly in place for this purpose.

Also as a poultice, it can be used for the relief of swollen, hardened breasts and mastitis – either chop the leaves up into a pulp, add a small amount of hot water, and apply as a thick pack, covered in muslin, or use the infused oil to make a salve. Apply the salve to muslin and place this on the affected breast or breasts.

Use as a mouthwash or gargle for sore throats and bleeding gums.

Rub the herb on the skin to repel biting insects – though given its name of "Stinky Bob", this might repel people as well!

It can be used as a hand or foot bath to help remove toxins, radiation and heavy metals from the system, and also to draw toxins from swollen lymph glands. Allow two well-chopped or shredded handfuls of leaves to a basin, cover them with boiling water and steep until the water is a comfortable temperature, then soak the hands or feet in it for 30 minutes.

Apparently it grows particularly abundantly in areas with high concentrations of radiation. The herb absorbs the radiation from the soil, breaks it down and disperses it. The whole plant repels deer and rabbits – perhaps one of the reasons why I have seen so few of either of these critters in my garden – just the odd hare, who is always welcome.

Folklore   There are three different bits of lore around the name. It is possibly named after a monk called Robert, who used it to heal many different disorders and complaints. Another legend reckons it is named after Puck, or Robin

Goodfellow – derived from Old English "Pucelas", or "Wild Men of the Woods". Plants named Robin have a traditional association with devils, death and the fae folk, and since I have a soft spot for all this sort of folklore, I much prefer this association myself!

Dose   Daily doses of 1 tsp (5 ml) of the tincture – but the strength of the tincture is not commonly agreed upon. I'd assume that this dose would be perfectly fine for a standard cottage-style tincture, made by just covering the dried plant material with vodka at 37.5% proof.

As a tea, it is often best as a cold infusion, probably because of the high volatile oil content – it would be a shame to evaporate off all those essential oils!

Contraindications   None known at present.

Herb robert recipes

Herb robert and plantain healing balm

Ingredients
- » ½ pint, loosely packed, of herb robert
- » ½ pint, loosely packed, of plantain leaves
- » sunflower oil
- » myrrh essential oil
- » frankincense essential oil
- » beeswax

Instructions   Finely chop the herbs and put them into the top of a double boiler, then cover with the sunflower oil. Put water in the bottom level and simmer gently over a medium heat until the oil has changed colour, then strain out the herbs. Add 12 g of beeswax per 100 ml (3½ fl oz) of oil and warm gently until the wax has dissolved; stir briefly, then add 5 drops each of myrrh and frankincense essential oils before pouring the salve into jars to set.

This balm is excellent for all sorts of minor cuts, grazes, bumps and bruises, and is a very handy thing to have a small pot of with you whenever you are out and about.

Herb robert, sweet cicely and self heal restorative tonic

Ingredients
- » ½ pint, loosely packed, of herb robert leaves
- » ½ pint, loosely packed, of sweet cicely leaves, and some of the sweet cicely green seeds as well
- » flowering self heal tops, gathered later in the summer
- » brandy or vodka
- » local honey or maple syrup

Instructions   As with many tonic recipes, finely chop the clean leaves and pile them into a Kilner jar, then pour over plenty of the alcohol – enough to cover the leaves with 5 cm (2 in) or more on top. Put the lid on and let the whole thing infuse for at least two months, until you see the first self heal flowering either in the garden or locally; then, add 1 pint, loosely packed, of finely chopped self heal flowers as well, stirring well and leaving the medicine to steep for another two weeks. Sweeten it to taste with maple syrup or honey – be sure you try it first, though, as sweet cicely has a sweet flavour, as the name suggests, so it may already be sweet enough. You can use dried self heal if you'd prefer: if so, add it at the same time as the fresh herb robert and sweet cicely, allowing around 100 g of it. Two weeks after adding the last batch of herbs, strain them out and bottle the resulting tonic. Take 5 ml three times a day to help you recover from illness or surgery, or just as a pick-me-up if you are feeling run down and exhausted.

Herb robert and ground ivy tonic for gut health

Ingredients

> ½ pint of loosely packed herb robert
> ½ pint of loosely packed ground ivy
> unpasteurised cider vinegar
> local honey or maple syrup

Instructions   Finely chop the herbs and pack them into a Kilner jar, then cover them with plenty of the vinegar, allowing an extra 2.5 cm (1 in) on top. Leave the whole lot to steep for a month, then strain out the herbs and sweeten to taste, shaking up the vinegar thoroughly afterwards to mix it well together. Add 10 ml of the tonic to 570 ml (20 fl oz) of water once a day and sip, to encourage better gut health.

Herb robert and ground ivy bladder and kidney tonic tea

Ingredients

> » herb robert, dried, enough for half a jar
> » ground ivy, dried, enough for half a jar
> » hot water

Instructions   To make a whole jar of this, gather the fresh herbs on a dry day when they are in full flower, making sure to pick only the healthy-looking stems. Pick the plants, stem and all, allowing at least 25 cm (10 in) per stem, if possible, though shorter ground ivy stems are fine as well. Make sure that the plants are clean and dry, then bundle them up with elastic bands before hanging them up to dry in a cool, dry room with not too much sun and good ventilation. Dried, the herbs should look quite similar to their fresh counterparts, just a lot smaller.

Once you are happy the plants are suitably dry, finely chop them using a pair of kitchen scissors or herb scissors. Often a food processor won't work for this sort of job as the stems, even dried, are still too flexible. Once the herbs have been thoroughly chopped into little pieces no bigger than 3 mm square, thoroughly mix them together and store them in an airtight glass jar. Label the jar carefully with the contents and instructions as follows: allow 1 tsp (5 g) of the herb per mug of hot water that is just off the boil. Cover the cup with a saucer, or make up the tea in a teapot or cafetiere. Let it steep for 5–10 minutes, then strain it and drink it hot. You can sweeten it to taste. If you really don't like the flavour, consider adding a slice of lemon or orange. Drink this tea once or twice a day as a tonic for the kidneys and bladder.

Jack-by-the-hedge
Alliaria petiolata

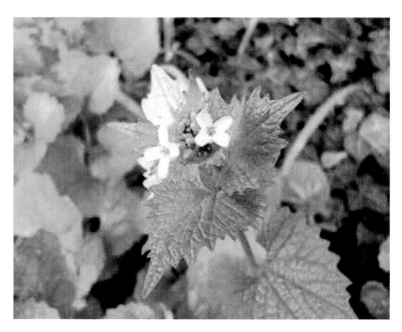

Also known as: garlic mustard, garlic root, garlicwort, poor man's mustard, sauce alone

Family Brassicaceae.

Habitat and description This pretty biennial is commonly found growing near hedges (as the name indicates) as well as tucked into flower beds, in verges and grassy areas, in wild lands and waste ground and around the base of trees. In the first year it produces a small clump of round, slightly pointed leaves that have a noticeable smell of garlic when crushed or torn. In the second year, it produces long stems with tiny white flowers on and leaves that begin translucent and touched with a faint hint of russet, and age into large green leaves marching up a tall, slender stem. The seeds are produced in long slender seed heads after flowering. The flowering stems can grow up to 1 m (3 ft) tall, towering above grasses and peeking out from between hedgerow plants.

Where to find it   Found across the UK and most of Europe, as far north as Scandinavia, and also as far afield as Morocco and other parts of Africa as well as America and western Asia.

Parts used   The young leaves and flowers, plus the tender stems.

When to gather   April and early May are best – the leaves go rather tough later on.

Medicines to make   Infused oils and balms for wounds, cuts and grazes. Salt blends, pestos and soups as food. Dried as a spice or seasoning for cooking.

Constituents   None really known at present as it really hasn't seen much research, but most likely volatile oils and compounds similar to those found in other members of the brassica family.

Planetary influence   Mars.

Associated deities and heroes   Most likely linked with deities associated with Mars, but possibly also with cooking and the hearth and home.

Festival   Beltane.

Constitution   Hot and dry.

Actions and indications   Not much used medicinally today, Jack-by-the-hedge has high levels of vitamin C and has been used as a diuretic and wound disinfectant. Far more often, the plant is used as a food, both cooked and raw; its vitamin C content can be helpful in boosting the immune system in the spring. The leaves can also be used internally, as a medicine to promote sweating.

Jack-by-the-hedge poultices have long been used on wounds, The fresh leaves can also be finely chopped, moistened and used topically as a poultice for bronchitis and chest issues, for bites and stings – where the plant can relieve the itching – and also as an antiseptic poultice on ulcers. It can also be included in infused oils for wounds, cuts and scrapes. To add an extra cleansing action; the root and leaves can be infused in oil as a chest balm or poultice for chest issues like asthma and bronchitis.

Folklore   This plant is one of the oldest known spices in Europe, with evidence of it dating back to 4100–3750 BCE. Historically, it has been used for flavouring salted fish, for extra flavour in soups and pottages, and mixed with other leaves as a salad.

The plant is considered an invasive species in parts of

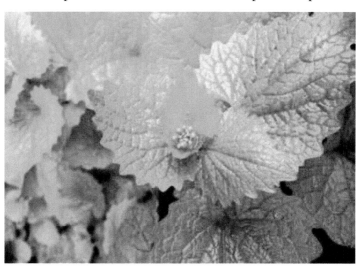

America, definitely giving an extra good reason for eating as much of it as you can! Make sure any plants you gather are free of pesticides and herbicides, and try to get the whole thing, including the root, which has a flavour rather like that of horseradish. This should at least stop the plant from quite taking over as much space as it is known for in the USA, where it crowds out many native and endangered plants. It's the usual case, really: it was taken there from the UK and has proved a nuisance ever since, in much the same way as ground elder and Himalayan balsam are a nuisance.

Dose   No particular dose is known – best eaten as a food, I think.

Contraindications   As with all members of the brassica family, use with care or avoid completely if you have thyroid issues.

Jack-by-the-hedge recipes

Jack-by-the-hedge butter

Ingredients / equipment
- » one handful of fresh Jack-by-the-hedge
- » herb salt
- » one large pot of double cream
- » one large empty Kilner jar with watertight lid

Instructions   Make fresh butter (see recipe above for dandelion butter). Once you have eliminated most of the buttermilk, take about 1 tbsp of really finely chopped Jack-by-the-hedge and mash it thoroughly into the butter, with a decent pinch of the herb salt. Taste a small amount. Add more salt, as needed. This will keep in the fridge for several days and can be used instead of garlic butter in cooking, or spread straight onto fresh bread.

Jack-by-the-hedge, dandelion flower and ground elder pesto

Ingredients

> » 1 pint, at least, loosely packed, of young Jack-by-the-hedge leaves
> » 1 pint, at least, loosely packed, of dandelion flowers without the green stems
> » 1 pint, at least, loosely packed, of young shoots of ground elder
> » 1 bulb of garlic or at least 3 large cloves
> » 125 g (4½ oz) of unsalted cashew nuts
> » olive or organic sunflower seed oil
> » salt

Instructions   Make sure your leaves are all clean, dry, and ready to use. If you have to use them damp, I strongly advise you use the resulting pesto as quickly as possible, as there is a risk that the extra water content could make the oil go rancid! Pull the yellow petals off the dandelion flowers and put them into a food processor, along with the other leaves, then add the cashew nuts, the peeled and roughly chopped garlic, and a good slosh of oil, then blend thoroughly. Add more oil until the pesto reaches the consistency you desire. Have a taste and, if you want, add some salt. Store in clean jars, with a layer of oil on top to preserve it a little longer, and keep in the fridge. This is lovely with fish or meat, as a topping for roasted vegetables, mixed into pasta, smeared onto fresh bread, or even dolloped onto salad!

Jack-by-the-hedge salt blend

Ingredients

> » plenty of fresh young Jack-by-the-hedge leaves
> » sea salt

Instructions Ideally you need a dehydrator for this, but an oven on the lowest setting with the door ajar should work as well. Check over the leaves for any bugs or marks, and then lay them out in a thin layer. If you are using a dehydrator, put the lid on once all the leaves have been spread out, and dehydrate on a low setting until the leaves are completely dry. If you are using the oven, check on the leaves every 10 minutes to begin with, to make sure that they aren't burning, then every half hour after that, until the leaves have become crisp and dry. Pile the dried leaves into a mortar and use the pestle to grind them into a powder, then add a roughly equal amount of sea salt. If you are using crystals, break those down in the mortar as well. If the salt is already in powder form, just mix the herbs in and pile the whole lot into a jar. This seasoning blend can be used in cooking, when making garlic mushrooms, sprinkled onto flatbreads, as part of salad dressings, or just sprinkled directly onto food: it is delicious. Provided water is kept out of the storage jar, it should last for months.

Wilted Jack-by-the-hedge and ground elder with lemon and butter

Ingredients
- » young, slightly translucent leaves and stems of Jack-by-the-hedge – at least ½ pint, loosely packed, per person
- » plenty of young stems of ground elder – at least ½ pint, loosely packed, per person
- » 1 large dollop of good-quality butter – I tend to suggest around 10 g per person
- » 1 organic lemon
- » salt – why not use the seasoning blend detailed above?

Instructions Check the leaves over carefully. In a frying pan, melt the butter until it just begins to sizzle, then pile in the herbs, stirring them regularly until they have wilted. Zest the lemon and add the finely chopped zest to the mixture, then squeeze over the juice of half a lemon and add enough salt to suit your preference. This is a lovely side dish to rich foods, where the herbal flavours and lemon provide a super contrast. Why not serve it alongside roasted sweet potatoes topped with homemade pesto?

Salmon or vegetables with crunchy Jack-by-the-hedge pesto topping

Ingredients
- » 1 salmon fillet per person; alternatively, a selection of vegetables – sweet potatoes, courgettes and peppers are lovely
- » home-made Jack-by-the-hedge pesto (see recipe above)
- » vegetable oil

Instructions   Lay the salmon on some baking foil or a silicone baking sheet and top it with a thick layer of the Jack-by-the-hedge, dandelion flower and ground elder pesto, making sure you cover the entire top of the fish. Bake in an oven set to 180°C for 25 minutes, until the salmon is fully cooked and the pesto is brown and crunchy. Eat immediately.

For the vegetable version, chop the vegetables into cubes or pieces and drizzle with plenty of good-quality vegetable oil before roasting with the oven set at 180°C until the vegetables have gone soft and have just begun to brown on top. Add the pesto at this point, smearing a generous layer over the top of the vegetables, and return the pan to the oven until the pesto is brown and crunchy. Eat without delay!

Lesser celandine
Ranunculus ficaria / Ficaria verna

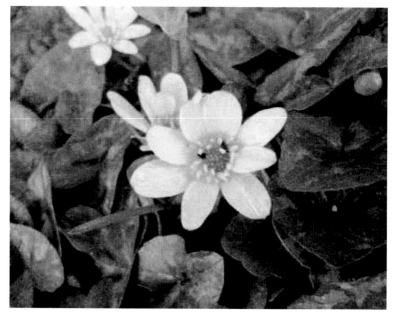

Also known as: pilewort, fig buttercup, figwort, smallwort

Family   Ranunculaceae.

Habitat and description   Appearing in early spring through to late summer, this low-growing perennial sports hummocks of quite thick, glossy bright-green leaves that are roughly kidney or heart-shaped and sometimes have darker markings on them. From February through to May, the plant is covered with bright-yellow flowers rather resembling buttercups, sometimes with a greenish tinge to the undersides of the petals. The whole plant likes to colonise damp, grassy areas, forming dense mats of growth full of glints of sunshine alongside white daisies and the ever-present dandelions. The roots form nodules under the ground in creamy oval clusters – a possible source of the folk name "pilewort"; they were used in the past, once thoroughly cooked, as a food source. However, the plant is generally held to be poisonous when ingested and should only be used externally.

Where to find it   Europe, Asia and North America, where it is considered a noxious weed.

Parts used   Roots and leaves.

When to gather   Spring and summer.

Medicines to make   Infused oils, balms, plaisters and poultices, predominantly for varicose veins and piles. Liniments and rubs for the same.

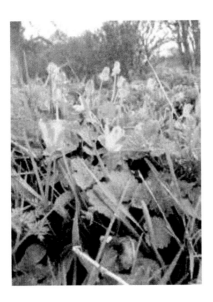

Constituents   Anemonin and protoanemonin, tannins, vitamin C and triterpenoids.

Planetary influence   Mars.

Associated deities and heroes   Sun deities – no surprise, really, given the beautiful flowers.

Festival   Ostara / Spring Equinox.

Constitution   Hot and dry.

Actions and indications   Lesser celandine is not widely used these days, but it can be used to make a balm, poultice or cream for haemorrhoids, as well as for varicose veins, as the whole plant is astringent, with some pain-killing and -soothing properties. The oil can also be used to formulate suppositories for piles situated further inside the anus.

Upon drying, the poisonous anemonin degrades to proto-anemonin, so it is more often used dried than fresh. Today, the plant is not used other than topically for haemorrhoids, though it could potentially be added to balms for varicose veins as well, because of its astringent properties. It is not used internally at all these days.

As a topical dressing it can also be useful in the treatment of abscesses. The roots can be dug up, cleaned and pulverised to form a treatment for stubborn varicose veins, abscesses and piles – apply as a poultice and leave it in place for up to an hour so that it can work its magic.

Folklore   Lesser celandine was called "pilewort" as the shape of the root nodule was thought to closely resemble haemor-rhoids. Wordsworth was particularly fond of the plant, and it is carved on his tomb. The Celts were also rather attached to celandine and named it "Grian", after the sun.

Dose   Internally not taken at all.

Contraindications   Do not take internally as it is poisonous.

Lesser celandine recipes

Lesser celandine balm for varicose veins and piles

Ingredients
- » 1 pint of loosely packed celandine leaves and flowers, as well as some roots, if possible
- » organic seed oil
- » beeswax

Instructions   Check over and finely chop the celandine – the roots need to be thoroughly clean, and if they are still rather soggy, put them on a sunny windowsill to dry out completely or wrap them in either kitchen paper or a clean tea towel and rub them vigorously to remove excess water. Put the herbs in the top of a double boiler and pour over the seed oil, until 1 cm of oil sits above the level of the plant matter. Warm the pan gently, until the oil turns green. Strain out the herbs and add 12 g of beeswax per 100 ml (3½ fl oz) of oil. Return the oil and wax to the top of the double boiler and warm the mix until the wax melts, stirring it regularly; then pour it into small jars. This strongly astringent balm can be used on varicose veins and piles, which is why no essential oils have been added. You can add herb robert and young horse chestnut leaves to this to really amplify the astringent, healing effects.

Lesser celandine poultice for abscesses and varicose veins

Ingredients
- » 1 small handful each of the leaves and flowers of lesser celandine
- » 1 or 2 of the small root nodules

Instructions   Make sure all the plant parts are clean, then chop them with a mezzaluna before putting them into a heavy, rough-sided mortar and using a heavy pestle to work them into a thick pulp. Add a tiny drop of water if you need to, to encourage it to hang together as a mush. This can then be scooped out of the mortar and packed onto a square of muslin. Apply the poultice to the abscess or varicose vein that needs particularly firm treatment, and lightly bandage it in place, leaving it for at least half an hour to work its magic. Remove it, wash off any excess bits of herb if need be, and leave it to dry in the open air.

Lesser celandine liniment

Ingredients
» plenty of fresh lesser celandine leaves, flowers and root
» vodka

Instructions   A liniment is basically plants preserved in alcohol – in this case, the vodka. Finely chop the checked and cleaned herbs and roots and pile them into a clean, dry glass jar, then pour over enough vodka to cover them. Put the lid on, and let it infuse for at least two weeks – four might be better, due to the inclusion of roots. Strain out the herbs at the end of this time and bottle the resulting liniment, making sure you label it with the name and date and "external use only". This liniment can be applied to a cotton wool pad and bandaged lightly over varicose veins, thread veins and similar issues for up to half an hour to encourage the veins to tighten back up.

Nettle
Urtica dioica

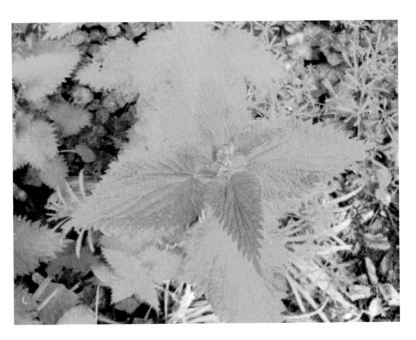

Also known as: stinging nettle, devil's apron, naughty man's plaything, tanging nettle, scaddie, hoky-poky, devil's leaf, heg-beg, jenny-nettle, sting-leaf, ortiga ancha, wergulu

Family   Urticaceae.

Habitat and description   Nettle really doesn't require much of an introduction or even a proper description, being well known by pretty much anyone who has ever been stung by it. Our friend the nettle grows in clumps that spread via the sturdy yellow roots, usually from a "queen" plant, with smaller clumps emerging in a circular pattern around the nettle matriarch. She grows up to around 150 cm (5 ft) tall in places and has a tough, ridged central stem, with opposite-paired leaves that are deeply toothed, dark green in colour, and with the characteristic hairs all over both the stems and the leaves. These hairs contain the formic acid that causes the pain when you brush up against the plant unwittingly. If you grasp a nettle firmly, she won't sting you – it is a light touch that causes the memorable discomfort of a nettle sting. Nettle grows in wastelands, woodlands, by the roadsides, in the middle of the vegetable patch – anywhere she can get her roots in, basically. Both greater and lesser nettles are found all over the UK, although in the USA the smaller nettle (*Urtica urens*) is found more commonly than the tall, lanky version we often find in the UK. *Urtica urens* is a much lower-growing version of our tall nettle, with a richer green colour to the leaves, which are also more deeply toothed, though both have similar medicinal virtues.

Nettle is harvested before the plant flowers, during March and April, if possible; however, it can be gathered at any time of the year for use as a liquid plant food, for which it combines beautifully with comfrey.

Where to find it   Europe, parts of North Africa and Asia, New Zealand and North America.

Parts used   Leaves, roots and seeds.

When to gather   Young shoots from February until late April, before the plant flowers. Roots in the winter months. Seeds from August onwards.

Medicines to make   Nettle tincture or syrup, nettle tea, nettle elixir, nettle-infused oil, nettle seeds for salads, soups, stews and smoothies, dried nettle. Add the leaves to soups, stews, pastas and breads. Dry and pulverise young nettles as a "seaweed" substitute in cookery. Seeds can be saved and used as an adaptogen or sprinkle.

Constituents   The root contains lignans, lectins, triterpenes and oleanolic and ursolic acid. The leaves contain flavonoids, glycoproteins, indoles including histamine and serotonin, assorted vitamins including vitamin C, fibre, iron, caffeic acid derivatives and protein.

Planetary influence   Mars.

Associated deities and heroes   Agni, Blodeuwedd, Hades, Horus, Cernunnos, Jupiter, Osiris, Pluto, Thor, Vishnu, Serpent deities and Vulcan. Nettle seems to be one of those odd herbs that caters equally to total opposites – sun and underworld deities. I don't personally associate it with Blodeuwedd, but some do – to each their own. The general consensus seems to be that nettle is a masculine herb, but I disagree: nettle has always felt feminine to me, but in a sharp, spiky,

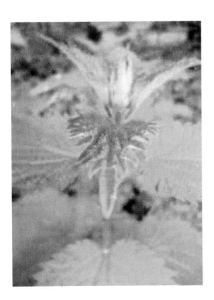

opinionated way. She's the older relative who chivvies you along, tells you to get on with it, get moving, do what you have to do. She quite literally stings you into action!

Festival I'm inclined to say Samhain, though it has associations with all the festivals. I tend to find that the typical "dark night of the soul" occurs between Samhain and Yule, and nettle is certainly a useful herb to allow perspective and clarity as well as to help you last through such trials and give you the stimulus necessary to encourage you to get moving and pull through when you feel bogged down.

Constitution Some say hot and dry, but I'd be more inclined to say neutral in a purely physical sense – though in a mental and emotional sense it certainly has got fiery aspects to it.

Actions and indications Our friend the nettle really deserves a much better reputation than the current one! A fantastic tonic herb, nettle has high levels of iron and can be taken by anyone who has problems with anaemia, and as a way to improve health in general. Nettles are best eaten as a tonic vegetable or used to make a fresh plant tincture, because many of the benefits are lost upon drying, though dried nettle is still a valuable health ally.

Due to their astringent, haemostatic properties, nettles are very good for haemorrhages and can be applied to wounds to stop bleeding, or taken internally to relieve excessive menstrual bleeding. They can also be used to relieve simple diarrhoea, enteritis and colic and are particularly recommended where mucus is present in the stool.

Nettles contain huge amounts of trace minerals, making them an important addition to any prescription aimed at improving mineral balance, and as part of prescriptions to improve resistance to allergies, asthma, eczema and hayfever.

As an extension of the herb's use to improve the body's resistance to hayfever, in cases of bronchitis and related problems it can also be taken to encourage the removal of phlegm from the respiratory tract. I've often also used it as a spring tonic, with chickweed, cleavers and dandelion root and leaf, to remove accumulated rubbish from the body caused by much inactivity over the winter snows. I'd be inclined to make a fresh nettle tea with added mild spices, as I am not over-keen on the flavour of nettle tea, though it can be made much more pleasant with the addition of ginger.

Nettles have a mildly hypoglycaemic effect, and can be used as part of a scheme to manage diabetes. It is a good tonic for the digestive system as a whole, especially where protein digestion is concerned. Some sources suggest its use for abnormally low blood pressure, to encourage it back to normal levels.

As a diuretic, it is used to relieve any health problems caused by an impaired ability to remove waste products from the body – in cases, for example, of gout and arthritis. It is a useful tropho-restorative, bringing the body back into balance. It has even been used to encourage the thyroid to regrow after surgery.

During pregnancy, nettle makes a fantastic iron tonic, and after birth it also encourages the production of breast milk. Later on in life, nettle is very good for women going through the menopause, as its high calcium content can help to ward off osteoporosis. Taken internally, nettle promotes healthy hair, skin and nails, as well as having a long-term beneficial effect on the overall health of the body. Used as a hair rinse, it leaves the hair shining and can relieve any scalp infections and problems.

In some cases of muscular atrophy, nettle has been very useful, especially for atrophy of the pelvic muscles and inner thighs in women – yet another good reason for pregnant women to take the herb!

Topically, a poultice of nettle leaf can be used to soothe the heat and inflammation associated with burns – nettle works very well alongside lavender and aloe vera for this. Another long-standing topical use of nettle is that of urtication, where you apply raw nettles to the skin in order to improve blood flow and circulation. This has been used to relieve arthritis and joint problems and to restore feeling to areas that suffer from numbness.

Nettle root can be used to relieve benign prostatic hypertrophy in men. The seeds have gained a reputation for healing the kidneys and have even helped some people to stop needing dialysis. Personally, I highly recommend nettle as an addition to the herbal first aid kit – it is easy to find, pick and make into medicine, has no contraindications, and is a valuable ally.

Nettle seed is a superb tonic for the kidneys and can be used to make a useful adaptogen. Gather the seeds and tincture them fresh for a more stimulant effect, or dry them for a more tonic adaptogen effect.

Nettle is a rather good food herb: it makes a wonderful soup or a delicious steamed green, with a flavour rather like spinach; it can also be added to pasta or gnocci for a hedgerow-themed slant to the evening meal.

Apart from making a superb liquid plant food, nettle is also a very good companion plant, improving the health of the soil and encouraging more healthy vegetables. It is particularly good as a companion plant to strawberries.

Folklore   A fairly large body of folklore surrounds the humble nettle, as befits such a widespread and useful plant. On the prosaic level, the stems yield a tough fibre that has been used by many different cultures to make clothes, ropes, nets and paper.

The nettle's name comes from the Latin word "uro", meaning "I burn" – appropriately enough, given how uncomfortable nettle stings seem to burn! Some think that the common name for the nettle comes from the Anglo-Saxon word "noedl", or needle, possibly referring to the tiny hairs that pierce the skin so easily and inject the acid that causes a nettle sting, or possibly referring to the plant's long use to make fabric.

Nettles have of old had an association with lightning, and with serpents. Legends say that the Great Serpent Lightning gave the plant some of his sting, while others speak of the Underworld Serpent giving the plant some of his poison. Romany gypsy folklore states that the nettle grows in places where there are underground passages to places where Earth faeries, or Pcuvus, dwell – the nettles are dedicated to these beings.

An old piece of lore from the venerable Albertus Magnus concerns the ability of nettles to attract fish when an infusion or oil of nettle and houseleek is applied to the hands. Apparently the fish swim gladly straight into the hand coated with such a preparation, though I rather suspect that if an oil were used, you wouldn't be able to hang on to the fish for long!

Dose   One tsp of the dried herb to a cup of hot water, three times a day. A tincture dosage of approximately 0.5–1.5 ml three times a day, as part of a prescription. I would probably not use more than 30 ml across a week's prescription – tea is a better way of taking the herb, to my mind, though it is a bit of an acquired taste.

Contraindications   None known at present.

Nettle recipes

Nettle syrup

Ingredients
- » 1 pint, loosely packed, of young nettle tops
- » lemon zest and juice of one lemon
- » spices, if preferred – cinnamon, ginger and star anise work well
- » brown sugar
- » at least 570 ml (20 fl oz) of water

Instructions Check over the nettle for bugs or bird poop, and rinse if needed. Chop them up finely, discarding any discoloured bits or any patches you aren't happy with, and put the finely diced herbs into a saucepan – enamel, stainless steel or glass is best; avoid aluminium, as it will leech into your remedy and really is not good for you. Add at least 570 ml (20 fl oz) of water per pint of herbs (prior to chopping them), and bring the whole lot to a gentle simmer. Add the lemon zest and juice, and any spices you wish to add (best to give these a bash with a mortar and pestle first, as these usually have a hard coating that makes it difficult for the water to get at them if they are not broken down first). Simmer the herb, spice and water mixture for at least 10 minutes to extract as much goodness as possible, then take off the heat and cool slightly.

Strain the liquid and herbs through a jelly cloth or clean piece of muslin and put the resulting fragrant liquid back into a pan. Add at least 500 g (1 lb 1½ oz) of sugar per pint (570 ml) of liquid – more is better, as it will preserve for longer. Honey unfortunately does not work for this kind of recipe, as it just doesn't preserve long enough when diluted with water. Return your pan to the heat and bring to a gentle boil, keeping a close eye on it – sugar burns very easily! Simmer the mixture gently until it has reduced down by about a quarter of the total volume. The consistency of the syrup should start to change about now, becoming thicker. Take it off the heat and pour it into clean bottles, capping it while still hot to get a good preservative seal on the bottle.

Nettle syrup can be taken year round to support the immune system and improve the body's ability to resist allergens in the atmosphere – ideal if you or a friend or loved one suffers from hayfever or allergies.

Nettle and spring green soup

Ingredients
- » 2 pints, loosely packed, of freshly picked young nettle tops
- » 1 large onion
- » 1 pint fresh watercress
- » 1 pint spinach
- » 1–2 pints in total, loosely packed, of other wild herbs, including fresh cleavers, chickweed, bittercress and jack-by-the-hedge if there is any around, in whichever proportions you can find
- » 1–2 pints (20–40 fl oz) of vegetable or herb stock
- » a dash of cream, if preferred
- » fresh garlic cloves – three or more

Instructions   Finely chop the onion and cook it gently in butter until it goes translucent. You can add lots of garlic at the same time if you love garlic – I certainly do, and will usually add around three cloves to this recipe. Wash and roughly chop or tear up the nettle, spinach, watercress and wild herbs and add it to the onion and garlic, stirring it around to mix it up thoroughly and begin wilting the leaves, then pour over the stock — at least 570 ml (20 fl oz), depending on how broth-like you want your soup. Simmer for a few minutes, until the leaves are fully cooked, then turn off the heat and use a stick blender to blitz until it is finely chopped. If preferred, add a dash of cream, and stir it in just before serving. Serve with good granary bread (homemade, with finely chopped nettle tops in, perhaps?) and fresh butter, or even with a poached egg on top of the soup. For a spicy kick, finish with plenty of freshly ground black pepper to make it a great warming lunch for chilly days!

Spiced nettle tea

Ingredients
  » 5 tbsp of dried nettle, or about 1 pint of fairly well-packed fresh nettle tops
  » approximately 570 ml (20 fl oz) of filtered water
  » zest and juice of 1 lemon
  » cinnamon
  » ginger (fresh and/or dried) to taste
  » cardamom pods
  » cloves
  » any other spices, as desired

Instructions   If you are using fresh ginger, peel and finely dice it, along with the zest of the lemon, then crush up any dried spices using a mortar and pestle until they are in fine pieces. Add all of your chosen spices, the lemon juice and the dried or fresh nettle to the water in a large pan. Bring the whole lot to the boil and simmer for 10 minutes; sweeten it as much or as little as you like, ideally using honey or maple syrup rather than sugar, then allow it to cool slightly. Filter it through a jelly bag and either drink it hot or allow it to cool right down.

This drink is high in vitamins and minerals, as well as containing the warming benefits of the spices! It will keep for three days in the fridge. Doses of up to three cups per day work well, and if you start drinking it fairly early, you will ward off much of the hayfever that is such a problem from about April onwards. You could also freeze this in ice-cube trays and add cubes to glasses of hot or cold water.

Spiced nettle and citrus syrup for hayfever

Ingredients
- » at least 1 pint of loosely packed nettle tops, or 50 g (2 oz) dried nettle herb
- » 1 large lemon
- » 1 large orange
- » 1 lime
- » spices to taste
- » 570 ml (20 fl oz) of water
- » 500 g (1 lb 1½ oz) sugar

Instructions Thoroughly chop the nettle leaves, and put them into a pan with the water and spices or syrup. Zest and juice the lemon, orange and lime and add these to the liquid, then bring the whole lot to a steady simmer. Simmer the concoction for 10 minutes, then filter out the herbs. Add the sugar, warm it over a low heat until the sugar has all dissolved, then bring it to the boil. Boil the mixture for 5 minutes, then take it off the heat and cool it slightly before bottling.

This can be taken in tablespoon doses to ward off hayfever, or diluted to make a hot or cold drink. Drink regularly to relieve hayfever and also symptoms of coughs and colds.

Nettle seed and lemon infusion

Ingredients
- » 1 tsp of nettle seed, ground – fresh is more stimulant, dried is more tonic
- » 1 slice of lemon
- » a little honey, if wanted
- » 1 cup of water

Instructions   Pop the ground nettle seed and slice of lemon into a pan with the water and simmer gently for 10 minutes, then strain out the herbs. Stir in a little honey if you prefer it that way, and drink slowly. If you are not sure how much nettle seed you can tolerate, start off with one tablespoon of the resulting infusion per day and gradually build up to one cup, either a whole cup in the morning or split the cup in half and drink half in the morning and half after lunch.

Nettle, pumpkin and sesame seed sprinkle

Ingredients
- » 2 tbsp, heaped, of nettle seed
- » 2 tbsp, heaped, of pumpkin seed
- » 2 tbsp, heaped, of sesame seed
- » pink Himalayan salt

Instructions   Using either a mortar and pestle or a coffee or herb grinder, roughly grind down the seeds until they are slightly coarser than powder consistency, then stir in the salt until the result is a texture and flavour you enjoy. Store it in a Kilner jar with a good, tight lid. You can sprinkle this on all sorts of foods: mix it into breads, shake it into salads, pour it onto roasted vegetables, meat or fish – use your imagination. This blend is rich in trace minerals and is also a great adrenal tonic.

Plantain

Plantago lanceolata / Plantago major

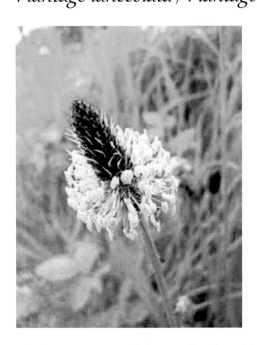

Also known as: Englishman's foot, broad-leaf plantain, cuckoo's bread, the leaf of Patrick, Patrick's dock, ripple grass, St Patrick's leaf, slan-lus, snakebite, snakeweed, waybread, waybroad (Anglo-Saxon, weybroed), white man's foot

Family Plantaginaceae.

Habitat and description Plantain is a low-growing perennial frequently found in hedgerows and by roadsides as well as in grassy meadows. It grows particularly well in earth that has been packed down by many people walking along it in all seasons – down on the common near where I used to live, there is a footpath that has been thoroughly trampled, and it is covered in plantain that grows where no other plant can manage; it has quite replaced the grass. There are two main kinds of plantain used medicinally – that I am covering in this profile anyway – and these are ribwort plantain (*Plantago lanceolata*), which has ovate, fairly long, thin leaves with deep veins, and broad-leaf plantain (*P. major*), which has much larger, broad, roughly oval-shaped leaves with the same familiar heavy veining.

The leaves themselves are juicy but tough. If you break a leaf, the central veins that run through the leaf will take more effort to break than the rest of the leaf. The leaves on both kinds grow in a central rosette, low to the ground, with the flowers appearing on long, slim, tough flower stems that grow to approximately 25 cm (10 in) tall. Ribwort plantain in flower is really a very pretty sight. The flowering heads, cream or pale pink in colour, are surprisingly eye-catching against green roadsides. For those with a whimsical imagination, like mine, they somewhat resemble miniature ballerinas. If you find any *Plantago media* – basically a cross between the other two varieties – the ballerina flower effect is even stronger!

Where to find it Europe, North America, parts of Scandinavia, parts of Asia; it is happy in most temperate climates.

Parts used Whole plant, especially the leaves.

When to gather April through September.

Medicines to make Plantain-infused oil and salve, plantain plaister, plantain elixir, plantain tincture, dried herb for tea-making.

Constituents Constituents found in plantain include iridoids; flavonoids such as aspigenin, scutellarin, nepetin and plantagoside; triterpenes; polysaccharides; plant acids such as fumaric and benzoic acid; fatty acids such as oleic acid and ursolic acid. It also contains trace minerals, including zinc, iron, calcium and sodium, as well as bitter compounds and vitamins A, C and K.

Planetary influence   Venus.

Associated deities and heroes   I have found none, much to my surprise, given that this is one of the nine sacred herbs of the Anglo-Saxons. It's possible that this herb can be associated with all deities and none, as a result of it being one of the sacred herbs, but this is pure speculation. Personally, plantain has always put me in mind of the Crone Goddesses, not so much because of its action but because of its strength and tenacity.

Festival   Not known.

Constitution   Cool and moist.

Actions and indications   Culpeper has quite a lot to say about this herb, after a short and rather pointed comment about the

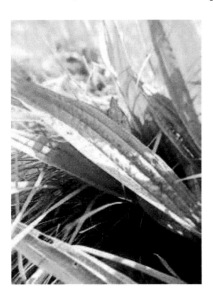

other astrologer physicians of his time regarding plantain as being ruled by Mars. His basic assessment of plantain is that it is astringent and soothing at the same time, being useful in the treatment of excessive loss of fluid from the body, whether this is in the form of excessive menstrual bleeding, or diarrhoea, or excessive urination. He also mentions that it is particularly good for lung problems such as ulceration and consumption, as well as being an excellent external agent for rheumatic complaints and gout, wounds, stings, bites and burns. Gerard has very little to say about the plant though, other than that the juice is good for cooling inflammation and infection of the eyes, which would seem to indicate more of an association with the moon than with Venus if you are paying attention to the astrological associations of plants.

In modern usage, plantain is indeed used to treat conjunctivitis; however, this is far from all of its uses.

The herb can be used to treat respiratory problems such as asthma and hayfever, as it has anti-asthmatic, antispasmodic, soothing properties that combine well with nettle. It can also be used to treat coughs, bronchitis, tuberculosis, and related inflamed conditions of the respiratory tract. It soothes and promotes the healing of inflamed, damaged respiratory surfaces, as well as being an expectorant, encouraging the removal of phlegm from the system. Several sources are of the opinion that ribwort plantain is the best plantain for the lungs, though I've heard mixed opinions about it. Either seems to work equally well. Use plantain either on its own or combined in equal parts with ground ivy (*Glechoma hederacea*) in large doses for sinusitis and related problems.

For the digestive system, it can bring ease to gastroenteritis, colic and related inflamed conditions of the digestive tract. It can also be used for chronic constipation, perhaps particularly for constipation due to lack of tone of the bowel muscles. The gently astringent, moistening properties of the herb will restore tone to the bowels. A tea of plantain leaves can be used to ease the discomfort of stomach ulcers and upset stomach, as it provides a soothing coating to the mucous membranes. The plant is excellent for removing toxins from the gut and for toning the digestive system.

It can be used to treat problems relating to the reproductive tract and urinary tract as well – as Culpeper mentioned – being useful in the treatment of excessive menstrual bleeding and inflamed conditions of the urinary tract, such as cystitis. It is used as a kidney tonic and to nourish and restore the whole urinary tract; it is particularly good for those with weakened systems that are prone to infection, and for those prone to incontinence.

Topically, plantain – especially broad-leaf plantain, *P. major* – has always had a good reputation as a wound healer. The fresh leaves can be picked and either chewed into a spit poultice or punctured repeatedly with the thumbnail and applied to wounds and stings to ease discomfort. The plant can be turned into a useful drawing ointment, which is applied thickly over the top of wounds with dirt in them or splinters, then loosely bandaged. The ointment will pull the muck out of the wound and draw the splinter out of the flesh. Other plants well suited for this use include marshmallow and slippery elm (in powder form).

Plantain is also an excellent herb for the mouth, great in the relief of inflamed gums and tooth infections. The tinctures can be used for this purpose as a mouthwash, or try a strong infusion or decoction of the leaves in the same way. The leaf, crushed and packed over the damaged area, can relieve pain and ease infection; I have also used it to great effect in the treatment of mouth ulcers and abscesses, where it can often draw out pus and encourage healing.

Folklore   The humble plantain is mentioned in the *Lacnunga* – one of the Anglo-Saxon medicine texts – as being one of the nine sacred herbs. It was used for poisonous bites and related injuries and was known as weybroed, because it grows on and near paths.

The name "white man's footstep" comes from the fact that it closely followed the new settlers to America and New Zealand, probably to the displeasure of the natives!

Plantain has been used in medicine for thousands of years, and has a reputation dating back to the Greek physicians.

Dose   A fairly strong infusion of the leaf can be drunk three times a day. Tincture dose for sinusitis works well at 10 ml up to four times a day. Combine it 50/50 with nettle as a hay-fever remedy and take 10 ml up to three times a day during particularly bad bouts.

Contraindications   None known at present.

Plantain recipes

Plantain and ground ivy allergy syrup

Ingredients
- » 1 large handful of plantain leaves
- » 1 large handful of ground ivy tops
- » 1 organic lemon
- » 570 ml (20 fl oz) of water
- » 500 g (1 lb 1½ oz) of sugar

Instructions   Finely chop the fresh herbs and put them into a pan with the water and the zest and juice of the lemon, then simmer it for a good 10 minutes. Filter out the herbs and put the liquid back into the pan with 500 g (1 lb 1½ oz) of sugar, warming it through until the sugar has dissolved.

Bring it to a gentle boil for 10 minutes, then pour into bottles and label it. Take one tablespoon of this morning and evening to relieve hayfever and related seasonal issues like rhinitis.

Plantain, thyme and eucalyptus chest salve

Ingredients
- » several large handfuls of fresh plantain leaves from the garden – either ribwort or broad-leaf is fine, or use a combination of the two
- » organic vegetable or seed oil
- » thyme essential oil
- » eucalyptus essential oil
- » beeswax

Instructions   Finely chop the clean, dry plantain leaves – you may want to give them a good bashing using a pestle and mortar as well, to really get the sap flowing. Pack them into the top of a double boiler, and pour over your organic oil. Rapeseed works well for this. Put the double boiler on a moderate heat and, keeping an eye on it, leave it to steep until the oil has changed colour to a deep, rich green: fresh leaves will give a darker colour than dry. You will then need to leave your resulting oil to settle for several hours, to allow any water to settle at the bottom; you can then carefully pour off the oil from the top, leaving the water behind. Once you have strained off the clear oil, return it to the pan, adding 10 g of beeswax to every 100 ml (3½ fl oz) of oil. Bring to a gentle warmth and stir until the beeswax has melted, then add 15 drops of eucalyptus and 5 drops of thyme per 100 ml (3½ fl oz) of oil, stirring and pouring immediately into jars. This balm can be applied to the chest, back, throat and the soles of the feet in the case of chest infections, coughs and colds.

Plantain, thyme and eucalyptus plaister

Ingredients

- » plantain, thyme and eucalyptus chest salve (see previous recipe)
- » clean muslin cloth

Instructions　There are two ways to make a basic plaister that I have used so far.

For the first method, I would advise making the plantain, thyme and eucalyptus chest salve with 15 g of beeswax per 100 ml (3½ fl oz) of oil, so that it melts more slowly.

Place a piece of clean muslin or other cloth (a quarter or a half of an old, clean cotton tea towel – waffle weave works well) into a bowl, and pour the hot salve over the top, allowing it to set; then pour another layer over the top to make a really thick layer. Take the cloth out of the bowl, use a spoon to scrape up any salve that has soaked through, and spread it on the top of the plaister. Once fully set, lay the whole thing on a large square of cling film – make sure it is about four times the size of the plaister itself – then simply fold one side of the cling film over to cover the plaister. Once that is done, roll it up like a large sausage roll and fold the ends in. This can be stored in a cool, dry cupboard until you are ready to use it.

For the second method, simply use a jar of your freshly made salve and, using a flexible knife or a spoon, scoop it out of the salve pot and smear it onto the cloth immediately before applying it to the skin. The disadvantage I have found to this method is that, as the salve does not have as much beeswax in, it melts a lot faster and can get rather messy!

When you want to use either sort of plaister for the chest or back, apply carefully to the affected area, cover with a layer or two of cling film wrapped around and over the top of the plaister and torso, then put a top over it. Lastly, apply a hot water bottle to the area to get the salve to soak in really quickly. If you are busy and unable to sit down for long enough, your own body heat will gradually melt the salve and get it to soak in.

Plantain tincture

Ingredients
  » plantain leaves – as many as you can gather!
  » spirits – vodka or brandy work well, the stronger you can get your hands on the better

Instructions   Partially dry your plantain leaves after checking them over, to remove at least half of the water content – this will allow your tincture to keep for longer. This can be done in a variety of ways: bundle them up and hang in a cool, dark place for a week or two, or layer them on a tray and put it in a very cool oven with the door open overnight, or use a dehydrator to quickly reduce the water content.

Once this is done, chop the leaves up finely – kitchen or herb scissors work really well for this. A knife and chopping board are not the tools for the job, as the drying process toughens the outside layer of the herb too much for the blade to slice through. Pack the chopped, dried herbs into a Kilner jar and pour brandy or vodka over them until it just covers the herbs. Press the herbs down thoroughly, put the lid on and leave it in a cool, dark place for a fortnight, shaking up regularly and then packing the herbs back down below the alcohol layer again.

Filter off the herbs and bottle the resulting tincture. I find this a really useful recipe for hayfever, to strengthen the lungs in cases of asthma, bronchitis, coughs and colds, and also for sinusitis. For the latter, I suggest you start with 10 ml twice a day, but in really acute cases try 10 ml four times a day for a couple of days, to really encourage the mucous membranes to soften up and regulate mucus production. A similar dose can be used for hayfever and bronchitis.

Plantain tincture, infusion, or decoction as mouthwash for mouth ulcers and abscesses

Ingredients
  » 6 medium to large plantain leaves

Instructions   To use plantain for mouth ulcers and abscesses, you can make an infusion or a decoction to use as a mouthwash. For the infusion, chop up enough fresh plantain leaves to allow 1 tsp, heaped, per cup of hot water. Pour over the water and leave the leaves to steep until cool, then strain out the herbs and use the resulting infusion as a mouthwash. Freeze the remaining infusion in ice-cube trays, so that you can take out one or two cubes for use each day.

Alternatively, you can use the tincture made in the previous recipe – allow 5 ml of plantain tincture to 5 ml of water, mix, and use as a mouthwash after brushing.

The decoction version is a little stronger than the straight infusion and can be made by boiling the herbs in the water until the water content has reduced by a quarter. Leave the leaves to steep until cool, then strain out the herbs and use the resulting infusion as a mouthwash. This mouthwash is great for inflamed, sore gums, whether through infection or abscess, or after dental surgery. The decoction, too, can be frozen, to be used as needed.

Plantain poultice for mouth ulcers and abscesses

Ingredients

  » 1–2 smaller plantain leaves

Instructions   To make a poultice for an inflamed, sore, abscessed or infected gum, make sure the plantain leaf chosen is clean, then cut it into pieces about 1 cm square. Pierce the surface thoroughly with a nail or a sharp knife, to ensure that the juices flow properly; if possible, put the pieces of leaf into a mortar and give them a few taps with the pestle to really break down the surface and get the juices exposed. Pack two or three squares treated this way between the infected gum and the side of the mouth, and leave there for half an hour each time, up to three times a day if possible, using fresh leaves each time. Follow up with a mouthwash of either plantain leaf or calendula and myrrh to encourage speedy healing.

Primrose

Primula vulgaris

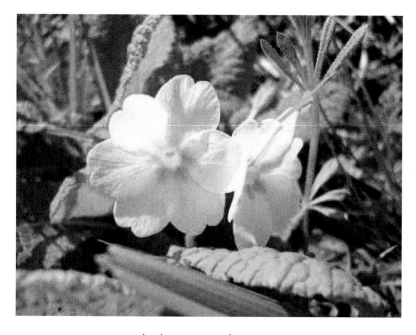

Also known as: butter rose, Easter rose, first rose

Family   Primulaceae.

Habitat and description   This lovely spring plant needs little description, really, as it is a common garden plant and can be found in increasing numbers in woodlands and by waysides! The leaves are roughly elongated oblong in shape. The young leaves emerge furled, so at first only the central stem can be seen; eventually they unfurl as they slowly grow. The flowers of the wild variety are a lovely sunny yellow, but there are now many beautiful cultivars available for purchase, in shades of pink through to rust colours. I do suggest that if you want to use this plant medicinally, go for the wild primrose, not the cultivars.

Be aware that cowslips and primroses have been considered endangered in the wild, and while the situation is improving, it is better not to harvest them in the wild unless you have a huge local patch and can gather enough for your medicine without damaging the plant population. My general rule of thumb is to make sure you can't see where you have been once you step away from the patch – other than the odd patch of bent grass, that is! The root should not be taken from the wild – why not consider growing your own instead, if at all possible?

Where to find it   UK and Europe, as well as further afield – many countries have their own version of *Primula vulgaris*.

Parts used   Leaves and flowers, root (dried).

When to gather   When in full flower – so generally in April. If you are taking the root, find 3-year-old plants in autumn.

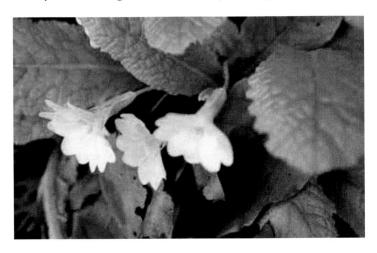

The leaves can be picked in April, but I have also gathered them as late as June if the plant has not yet finished flowering.

Medicines to make   Elixirs, tinctures, teas, infused oil, skin wash.

Constituents   Saponins, phenolic glycosides and flavonoids.

Planetary influence   Venus.

Associated deities and heroes   Freya, Blodeuwedd, any spring goddesses.

Festival   Ostara.

Constitution   Warm and moist.

Actions and indications   In many cases, primrose can be used interchangeably with cowslip, so do also check the information for that plant. As it is considered milder than the cowslip, it may be more useful for children.

In the past it was much used for rheumatism and gout, to relieve insomnia, and as a wound healer. A wash of the whole herb can be used to ease many skin problems, including acne and spots.

Primrose and cowslip both have a bit of an affinity with the nervous system and have been used to relieve nervous headaches and insomnia, as well as to settle anxiety, relieve panic attacks and ease mania.

As with cowslip, it can be used to relieve chesty coughs and bronchitis, but be aware that larger doses are emetic, so use small doses only.

Culpeper used the whole plant to make a wound healer that he considered one of the best he knew of, so why not use it to make a healing balm?

Folklore   Both the primrose and the cowslip are linked with fairyland, or the otherworld, as a variety of pieces of folklore from Germany and other European countries speak of a gate into fairyland being opened when a child placed a certain number of cowslips on a rock. She entered to find a castle and treasures awaiting her. When she was returned to her family later that day, an old miser who had watched her enter and then emerge with pockets full of gold tried the same trick, but he didn't use the right number of flowers. He was never seen again.

Primroses and cowslips have long been used to make a wash to increase beauty.

Dose   One teaspoon of flowers and leaves to a cup of hot water to make a tea, drunk twice a day; 5 ml twice a day of the tincture or elixir.

Contraindications   Too much primrose can cause nausea and vomiting, so start with a small dose and build up from there.

Primrose recipes

Primrose and plantain wound balm

Ingredients
- » 1 pint, loosely packed, of primrose flowers and leaves
- » 1 pint, loosely packed, of fresh plantain leaves
- » organic seed oil
- » beeswax
- » German chamomile essential oil

Instructions   As with all balm and infused oil recipes, check to make sure the flowers and leaves are clean and as dry as possible. If there is still moisture on them, as is fairly common with herbs gathered in the spring, dry them as much as possible with a clean cloth or some kitchen paper, then finely chop the herbs and pack them into a double boiler. Pour over enough seed oil to cover the herbs, allowing an extra 1 cm on top, then put the mixture on to heat through gently. Leave it until the oil has turned a rich jewel green, then strain the mixture through kitchen paper or clean muslin before adding 12 g of beeswax per 100 ml (3½ fl oz) of oil. Pop the oil and wax back into the cleaned double boiler, then put it back on the heat, stirring until the wax has melted. Add 10 drops of chamomile essential oil per 100 ml (3½ fl oz) of oil mixture, stir briefly to ensure it has mixed in properly, then pour the resulting balm into glass jars, put the lid on, and label them carefully with the name and date of production. This balm can be really soothing when used on cuts and grazes, bites and stings, and on dry, cracked skin.

Primrose and cowslip flower elixir for anxiety and insomnia

Ingredients
> » 1 pint, loosely packed, of primrose and cowslip flowers and leaves
> » brandy
> » local honey or maple syrup

Instructions   Finely chop the clean flowers – this time you don't need to worry whether they are surface dry. Pack the resulting herbs into a Kilner jar and pour over enough brandy to cover the plant matter, allowing enough honey to suit your taste. I find that 1 tsp (5 g) of honey per 100 ml (3½ fl oz) of brandy is usually a pleasant proportion; if you prefer your elixir sweeter than this, then tailor the recipe to suit your preference. Stir up the mixture until the honey has dissolved and mixed in, then leave the whole lot to steep for at least a fortnight. At the end of this time, strain out the herbs, bottle the elixir, and take 5 ml for anxiety, or two doses of 5 ml through the course of the evening for insomnia.

Primrose, cowslip and thyme cough syrup

Ingredients
- » 1 pint, loosely packed, of primrose and cowslip flowers
- » 1 tbsp of freshly picked thyme leaves
- » 570 ml (20 fl oz) of water
- » 1 organic, unwaxed lemon
- » 500 g (1 lb 1½ oz) sugar

Instructions   Finely chop all of the herbs; remove the zest from the lemon and chop it thoroughly. Put the herbs, lemon zest, lemon juice and water into a large pan and bring to a simmer, keeping a lid on it to keep the volatile oils in the saucepan. Simmer the mixture for 10 minutes, until the water content has reduced down by a third, then remove it from the heat and strain out the herbs through a sieve. This is a basic decoction, which can be taken as it is in 20-ml doses; if you would like to sweeten it, you can return the liquid to the cleaned-out saucepan along with 500 g (1 lb 1½ oz) of sugar, bring it back to a simmer, and stir until the sugar has dissolved. Bring the syrup back to a rolling boil, keeping a close eye on it, and boil it for 5 minutes until it begins to thicken. Remove it from the heat, cool it slightly, and bottle it hot, putting the lid on straight away and labelling it once the bottles have cooled – labels often won't stick to hot bottles. Take 10 ml up to four times a day to relieve coughs and chest infections. This mixture will store in the fridge for up to 6 months.

Sweet woodruff
Galium odoratum / Asperula odorata

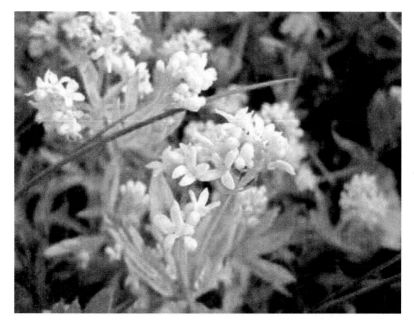

Also known as: wuderove, wood-rova, master of the woods,
masterwort, star grass, cordialis, musk of the woods, heart's delight

Family   Rubiaceae.

Habitat and description   This is one of my favourite herbs
in the wild garden, where it grows happily underneath the
largest of my apple trees. Woodruff is a rather beautiful little
perennial; if left to its own devices, it sprawls merrily over
increasingly large amounts of ground, drowning out even the
perennially thuggish buttercups. It produces a profusion of

slender, squarish stems up to 30 cm (12 in) tall, set about with slender, lanceolate leaves in whorls that march up the stem. The flowers, which open in May and June, are small and white, each with four petals. They smell wonderful: it is the coumarin content that is responsible for a fragrance that resembles that of new-mown hay and vanilla, making it a wonderful plant to bring inside for drying, which intensifies the scent. The plant spreads by way of creeping stems and roots, beginning as a small clump and forming large mats of growth – a lovely plant for the wild garden or for tucking underneath wooded areas, where there is too much shade for many other plants. It will also grow happily under hedges and in any area with less sun than most plants would find favourable. The seeds, when formed, are hard, rough little balls, a little like those of its cousin, cleavers; they will happily stick to any animals or other pedestrians that may pass, which allows the plant to propagate itself readily.

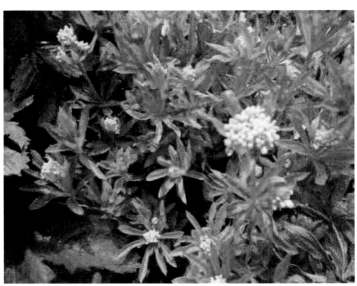

Where to find it   Woodruff is found in most of Europe, even in colder parts of the continent, including Siberia; it is also found in parts of Asia. The plant is naturalised in North America, where it can often be found growing in woodland.

Parts used   The aerial flowering parts.

When to gather   May and June, when in full flower.

Medicines to make   Sleep pillows, balms and infused oils, perfume oils, teas, decoctions, cottage tinctures.

Constituents   Coumarins, iridoid alkaloids, flavonoids and tannins, and anthraquinones, nicotinic acid, and asperuloside.

Planetary influence   Mars, according to some, but I personally link it more with Venus. I think it really depends on which aspect of the plant you are most focused on.

Associated deities and heroes   War deities like Mars; also faery folk linked with woodlands and deep forests and Beltane.

Festival   Beltane (no surprise there, really).

Constitution   Warm and dry.

Actions and indications   Woodruff is actually a surprisingly versatile plant with a wide array of possible uses and benefits, though I suspect the presence of coumarins has rather put many off its use. For the veins and circulation, the plant is anticoagulant, anti-inflammatory and a venous tonic, making it rather well suited to the relief of thrombophlebitis and phlebitis. It also acts as a blood thinner, removing blockages, improving varicose veins and getting the blood moving in the case of stasis and congestion. It opens up and supports the circulation and encourages the relaxation of tension in blood vessel walls in the case of stress-related hypertension. It has also been used to strengthen the heart, and I think it would combine well with hawthorn berries and flowers to make a delicious elixir for this purpose. The presence of coumarin has caused some concern in the past, but as far as I can tell it does not break down to dicoumarol, which is where blood thinning issues arise. In any case, do not take if you are on warfarin or similar blood-thinning medication.

In addition to this, the antispasmodic properties are also linked with the nervous system, giving the plant some handy properties in the relief of insomnia, anxiety and stress, as well as ameliorating panic attacks as part of a blend with herbs such as chamomile and lemon balm, and in the relief of migraine, particularly where there is a distinct link with the circulatory system, neuralgia, restlessness and depression. The plant can be used as a nervous restorative, but do monitor blood pressure while you are using it to ensure there are no problems with it.

Topically, the plant makes a lovely fragrant infused oil and balm suitable for cuts and wounds, and also for chilblains when combined with wintergreen essential oil.

As an aromatic, the plant can improve the digestive tract, as it is a fragrant and soothing stomach tonic and has some gentle antispasmodic effects on the liver as well. A small amount of the cold infusion can be used for heartburn, and the whole plant can relieve dysentery and constipation, again where there is spasm in the lower digestive tract walls.

Combined with other gentle bladder tonics, woodruff can be used to simulate the bladder and kidneys and to improve blood flow to these organs.

Lastly, as it is antispasmodic and calming, woodruff can be very useful for menstrual and menopausal issues, in particular in the relief of dysmenorrhoea or painful menstruation. Combine it with lemon balm (*Melissa officinalis*) and possibly cramp bark (*Viburnum opulus*) in this case. It can be used to ease the transition through the menopause as well, possibly when added to a motherwort elixir. Do monitor the plant's use in the case of excessive menstrual bleeding though, as it may make this issue worse due to its blood vessel relaxant properties.

Some hold that a cold infusion is to be preferred over a hot one – add 1 tsp of chopped fresh flowering herb to a cup of cold water and leave it to infuse overnight. Drink half-cup doses up to four times a day, no more than this. If you are using the dried herb, allow 1 tsp of chopped herb to a cup of water that is hot but well off the boil, cover it and allow it to steep for 5 minutes, then take half of a cup up to four times a day.

Folklore   The name "wood-rova" is thought to derive from the French "*rovelle*" or wheel, alluding to the spokes of the leaves as they surround the stem. The plant used to be used to stuff mattresses and strew on the floor, as it deters many of the smaller biting insects. The plant, when worn tucked into the helmet, has also been linked with battle prowess and success in battle.

In Germany, it is used to make infused wine drunk during May celebrations on the first day of May. The old name *Waldmeister*, "Master of the Woods", came from the plant's tendency to colonise the ground layer in woodlands.

Dose   One tsp (5 g) of dried sweet woodruff leaves, or 7.5 g of dried leaves, to a cup of hot water, infused for 5 minutes; take half a cup three to four times a day. Of the cottage tincture, start out with small doses of 1 ml in 10 ml water and sip slowly, mindful of the fact that larger doses can give you a queasy stomach.

Contraindications   Large doses can cause vomiting and dizziness. Do not use if you are on warfarin or other blood thinners.

Sweet woodruff recipes

Sweet woodruff sleep pillows

Ingredients / equipment

» plenty of dried sweet woodruff
» cotton material
» needle and thread
» fabric scissors

Instructions   First, you will need to dry plenty of sweet woodruff. This is best done on a sunny day when it is in full flower,
and you will need to pick fairly carefully, as the whole stem
including the root pulls free of the ground very easily. Use a
thumbnail at the base of the stem to nip it off, and gather the
herbs into either a basket or a soft cotton bag if it's a windy
day. Bring in the herbs and lay them out in a thin layer, in
baskets or on wide, shallow hydroponic drying trays, and leave
them for at least a week in a cool, well-ventilated room, until
they are fully dry. You'll know they're ready for use when they
have shrunk by about half and turned a more muted green.
They should be much more strongly aromatic at this point.

Use kitchen scissors to cut the woodruff into small pieces –
no longer than 1.25 cm (½ in), smaller if possible. Decide how
large you would like your sleep pillow to be and cut out a rec-
tangular piece of the cotton fabric you have chosen. Fold it in
half, with the pattern inwards if you are using patterned fabric,
then sew small, tight stitches along two sides, leaving one side
open. Turn the pouch the right way out, with the pattern fac-
ing outwards, and use the needle hooked into the corners to
pull them out if need be. Stuff the pillow thoroughly with
the dried, chopped woodruff, then turn the rough top edge
inwards and sew carefully along that edge as well. The pouch
should be slipped into a pillow case: it will flatten down fairly
quickly. You may want to change out the herbs each spring

for a fresh batch, depending on how strong the fragrance of the herbs still is.

May wine

Ingredients
- » 1 bottle of medium white wine
- » one bundle of fresh sweet woodruff in flower – five short stems is plenty
- » 4–5 clusters of hawthorn flowers
- » 2 lemon balm tops
- » maple syrup, if preferred

Instructions   Tie the woodruff flowers and the lemon balm tops into a bundle with a piece of cotton thread and pop them into a Kilner jar with the hawthorn flowers, then pour the bottle of white wine over the top. Put the lid on and put the jar into the fridge to steep; later that evening, decant it through a sieve and pour the resulting wine into a pretty jug. Serve as part of the May Eve celebrations.

Sweet woodruff tea blend for menstrual pain

Ingredients
- » 1 part dried lemon balm (e.g. 10 g)
- » 1 part raspberry leaf (e.g. 10 g)
- » 2 parts of dried rose petals (e.g. 20 g)
- » ½ part dried sweet woodruff (e.g. 5 g)
- » dried ginger – 1 tsp (5 g)

Instructions   Ensure that all the herbs are finely chopped, and mix them well together. Add the dried ginger (if using less of the main ingredients than listed, use ½ tsp of ginger), mix it well, and pile the whole thing into a clean, airtight jar. Label it

with the contents and ingredients, plus some instructions. Add
1 tsp (5 g) to a mug of hot water, cover the mug with a plate
and let it steep for 5 minutes. Sweeten the tea as you prefer,
and drink it up to four times a day to relieve period pain.

Double-infused woodruff and wintergreen balm

Ingredients
  » at least 2 pints of fresh or dried sweet woodruff, gathered
    while in flower
  » organic seed oil
  » beeswax
  » wintergreen essential oil

Instructions   Make sure that your woodruff is surface dry if
you have picked it fresh – if it is still a little damp, you may
want to lay it out in a tray and let it dry thoroughly overnight
before you begin making your infused oil. Once the fresh
herb is dry, or if you are using dried herb, finely chop it using
kitchen scissors, and pack half of it into the top of a double
boiler, covering the herbs with enough oil to allow an extra
0.5 cm of oil on top of the herbs. Put the double boiler onto
a moderate heat to slowly infuse the oil and leave it to steep
for at least an hour, two if possible. After this time, strain
out the first lot of herbs and replace it with a second round
of the chopped herbs, repeating the process. Strain out the
herbs again, and allow 12 g of the beeswax to each 100 ml
(3½ fl oz) of infused oil, returning both ingredients to the
cleaned top of the double boiler. Warm the oil mix until the
wax has melted thoroughly, then stir before adding 6 drops of
wintergreen oil per 100 ml (3½ fl oz) of the oil and wax blend.
Stir it all briefly, then pour into clean, dry jars and rest the lids
on top to stop the essential oils from evaporating. Once the
balm has set, seal the lids on tightly and label the jars with

the name and purpose of the balm plus the date when it was made. Apply the balm to chilblains and rub it well in.

Woodruff and southernwood moth-repellent sachets

Ingredients / equipment
- » dried sweet woodruff leaves
- » dried southernwood leaves
- » pinking shears
- » fabric pencil or chalk
- » cheesecloth or other loosely woven muslin-type fabric
- » cotton yarn

Instructions   Ensure that you have roughly equal proportions of dried woodruff and southernwood, perhaps 50 g (2 oz) of each, and finely chop them using clean scissors (not the pinking shears – those are for later!) Using the fabric pencil or chalk, draw around a clean small side plate onto the muslin fabric and use the pinking shears to cut out the circle. These kinds of scissors are great for removing the need to hem and stitch the sachets and are well worth having to hand if you plan to make this sort of thing regularly – you can find them in most dressmaking or haberdashery stores, or buy them online. They shouldn't be expensive.

Cut out at least four of the fabric rounds and pile a little heap of the chopped herbs in the middle of each one – allow about one handful of herbs per pouch. Draw up the sides, and cut a length of cotton yarn that is at least 38 cm (15 in) long. Fold the yarn in half and put the midpoint against the pouch, then wrap it tightly around two or three times before tying a tight bow in it. Use the loops of the bow to hang the sachet from a clothes hanger, or use it to scent clothing drawers.

Violet
Viola odorata

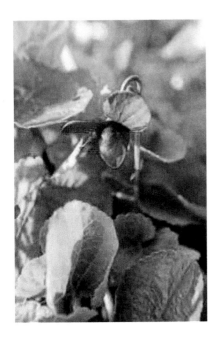

Also known as: English violet, sweet violet, blue violet, bairnwort, blaver, banwort, apple leaf, bessy banwood, vilip, cookoo's shoe, sweetling, garland flower

Family   Violaceae.

Habitat and description   The sweet violet is a low-growing perennial favouring roadsides, meadows and shady wooded edges. I have found it growing under huge walnut trees, among long grass, and dotting the roadsides in my home county of Lincolnshire, in a whole spectrum of blue shades, ranging from the traditional dark violet through to pale lilac and white. The leaves are a rich, bright green and are heart-shaped, with lightly toothed edges, staying fairly low growing to the roots. The whole plant does not generally grow more than about 12–15 cm (5–6 in) high, so you have to look quite carefully for it, as it is easily missed and rapidly gets swamped by grasses and taller plants as spring progresses. The flowers are fragrant, but only if you are close enough to the plant to pick up the elusive scent, and it fades quickly after the plant has been pollinated. The blue-purple flowers so often seen are actually not the reproductive flowers of the plant – those are small, green affairs that are very easily missed and are produced by the plant after the blue flowers have finished. It is generally the sweet violet, or its cousin, heartsease (*Viola tricolor*), that are used in medicine.

Where to find it   Europe and Asia, and it is naturalised in North America and Australia.

Parts used   The leaves and flowers.

When to gather   March, April and May.

Medicines to make   Violet-infused oil, elixir, or tincture. Dried leaves and flowers for tea. Candied violets.

Constituents   The plant contains quite a wide variety of con-stituents (no surprise there, all herbs do!), including, but not limited to: phenolic glycosides such as gaultherin and salicylic acid methyl ester (which may explain the anti-inflammatory action); volatile oils, including curcumene and zingiberene; saponins such as violin; flavonoids such as rutin and violaru-tin, and lots of mucilage.

Planetary influence   Venus.

Associated deities and heroes   Unsurprisingly enough, given some of its nicknames, the violet is associated with the love Goddesses Aphrodite and Venus, as well as with Io and Orpheus, and Aphrodite's son Priapus.

Festival   Ostara, the Spring Equinox, and Beltane.

Constitution   Cool and moist.

Actions and indications   The pretty, delicate sweet violet has quite a wide array of medicinal uses, including in treating problems of the lungs, digestive tract and nerves. As it is a cooling, moistening herb, it is predominantly used to cool, soothe and relax inflamed, over-stretched tissues.

It can be used to treat catarrh, coughs and colds, especially where these are long-lasting and deep-seated, as well as bronchitis, pleurisy and tuberculosis due to the saponin content of the herb, which promotes expectoration or the removal of phlegm from the lungs. It makes a fantastic syrup for soothing children's coughs and is useful for those suffering feverish colds, making it suitable for relieving the symptoms of influenza. It can be gargled to relieve sore throats and used as a mouthwash to treat inflamed, sore gums. It combines well with vervain and coltsfoot in the relief of whooping cough.

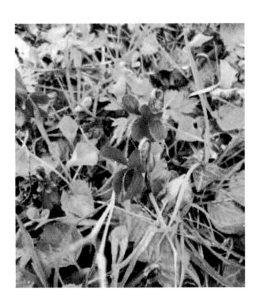

It is also a useful digestive herb and can soothe haemorrhoids and ease mild constipation and liver-related problems, such as jaundice. I would think that this is particularly applicable for overheated, tense people who anger easily and who are very stressed, but this is a theory at present.

As a soothing diuretic, it is useful in the relief of inflamed and painful urinary infections, such as cystitis and urethritis.

Violet has quite a reputation as an anti-cancer herb, with reports that an infusion of the leaf can ease cancerous pain. The root is emetic and should be used with caution.

It is said to improve the memory and moderate anger and can be of use in the relief of headaches and migraines, especially where there is a sensation of heat related to this. Sweet violet is a blood cleanser, so can be of use in the treatment of skin conditions such as eczema, both internally and externally. Topically, it can be used to treat skin inflammation. It is also antiseptic, antibacterial and antiviral and can be used as a cardiac tonic. As part of a long-term prescription, it can be used to help to relieve rheumatism and related inflamed joint conditions.

Folklore There's quite a wide body of folklore surrounding this flower, as its use and popularity dates back to the Greeks. The name "viola" is derived from the Greek name for the plant, "*ione*", named after Io, the daughter of Inachus, a river deity. Typically enough, Zeus took a fancy to her and decided to try to seduce her. He changed himself into a cloud in the hope that Hera wouldn't figure out what he was up to and approached Io — but, unfortunately for him and fortunately for Io (Zeus does not have a reputation for using gentle seduction methods, shall we say!), Hera was right behind him and turned Io into a white heifer. Zeus provided the heifer with a field of violets to eat. One has to wonder whether perhaps Hera was as annoyed at Zeus's womanising ways as she was saddened by the way he used and disposed of his lovers, not all of whom were willing. Then again, this is the same bad-tempered Goddess who became suspicious of the beautiful heifer in the field and sent flies to attack her, and the poor creature had to jump into the Ionian sea to escape them. She was turned back into a woman after Zeus had given his solemn promise never to look at her again.

The association the violet has with Orpheus comes from the myth that the plant grew where Orpheus's lute fell after the Maenads killed him. Zeus placed his lute in the heavens as a constellation, and the flower was dedicated to Orpheus. A different variation on this story states that the violets grew underneath the lute whenever Orpheus put it down. I have to admit, I prefer this story – with so much death and destruction in the Greek myths, it is pleasant to read a myth where someone hasn't died!

The Romans and Greeks both believed the violet to be a symbol of love, and both races liked to drink violet wine: amusing, considering that the belief that wearing a crown of violets would also cure a headache caused by over-indulgence in alcohol. I suppose it could be considered a metaphorical "hair of the dog that bit you"!

In the medieval era the violet was much loved: it was added to pot-pourri and was used to perfume linens and to flavour meads and alcoholic drinks, as well as both sweet and savoury dishes. Monks grew violet lawns, as somewhere fragrant to sit and meditate.

The violet was one of Queen Victoria's favourite flowers and was sold on the streets in London as well as being used extensively in the perfume industry at the time.

More recent folklore and history mention that Napoleon gave violets to his wife on each wedding anniversary, and they were used as his emblem and password when he was in exile.

Dose   1 tsp of the dried herb infused in a cup of hot water for up to 15 minutes, three times per day. Make sure you cover the cup, so you don't lose all of those lovely volatile oils in the steam. Dosage is roughly 2 ml of a 1:5 40%-strength tincture three times a day.

Contraindications   None known at present. The root can be emetic, so it is best not to use this part of the plant at home.

Violet recipes

Violet syrup

Ingredients
- » 1 pint of loosely packed violet leaves and flowers of the scented type of violet (*Viola odorata*)
- » 570 ml (20 fl oz) of water
- » 500 g (1 lb 1½ oz) – at least – of sugar

Instructions   Using a sharp knife, a mezzaluna or a food processor, finely chop the violet flowers and leaves, checking first for livestock or bird poop. Remember to pick your violets only in places where there is no crop spraying and the likelihood of dog mess is slim to none.

Having a patch of violets in your garden is ideal if you don't have any pets; otherwise check at the edges of woods and under hedges next to paddocks and suchlike. Once you have chopped the violet leaves and flowers, pop them into a pan (not an aluminium one) and add the water. Bring the mixture up to a gentle simmer and allow it to cook for at least 10 minutes, until the water has turned a deep blue-green colour. The syrup will smell a little like cabbage – rather sad, given the delicate fragrance of fresh violet flowers – but the resulting medicine doesn't taste too bad at all.

Once you have simmered the liquid for a good while and the amount of water has reduced down by one quarter, take it off the heat and filter out the herbs. Pour the liquid back into the pan with an equal amount of sugar – if, for example, you have 400 ml (14 fl oz) of decoction left, add 400 g (14 oz) of sugar. You can use less than this, but be aware that the resulting syrup will not keep for as long and will probably need to be frozen in ice cubes in order to preserve it.

Stir the liquid over a low heat until the sugar has dissolved, then simmer until it has started to thicken. Pour it into clean glass bottles and put the lids on while it is still hot, in order to get a good seal and encourage the syrup to keep for longer.

A good dosage of the syrup is 1 tbsp (15 ml) three times a day for coughs with raised lymph glands, and a similar dose for those experiencing unusual flares of anger with no discernible cause, which are out of character. If you are using it for the latter purpose, I strongly recommend some journalling as well, in order to pinpoint where the anger has come from.

Violet cooling elixir

Ingredients
- » ½ pint, at least, of violet leaves
- » ½ pint, at least, of violet flowers
- » rose petals
- » hawthorn flowers
- » honeysuckle flowers
- » vodka
- » maple syrup or local runny honey

Instructions   This is one of those recipes that you will need to work on in stages as the seasons progress, beginning with the violet leaves and flowers picked in April and May. Gather at least ½ pint of the leaves and ½ pint of the flowers and chop them finely before piling them into a Kilner jar and covering them with vodka, allowing an extra centimetre on top. Later, in May and early June, you can add hawthorn flowers and then, later still in the summer, you can add rose petals and honeysuckle flowers, finely chopped. Ensure that the vodka covers all of the herbs, topping it up if need be. Add the honey when you add the final batch of herbs, allowing 1–2 tbsp (up to 30 ml) of runny honey, more if you prefer. Let the whole elixir steep for at least a fortnight after the inclusion of last herbs, then strain out the plant matter and compost it. The resulting elixir can be taken in 10-ml doses up to three times a day to moderate excessive heat when this presents as a short, explosive temper, which I tend to think of as "liver heat", particularly when it is accompanied by redness in the face and a red tongue. It is particularly good for those who are generally quite calm and for whom an explosive temper is uncharacteristic. I often use this elixir and others like it in the summer for heat headaches, as well as for headaches linked with tight blood vessels and too much heat in general.

Violet and calendula mouthwash

Ingredients
- » plenty of violet flowers and leaves – up to ½ pint, loosely packed, if at all possible
- » fresh calendula flowers (later in the season)
- » vodka – the strongest you can find

Instructions   Finely chop the herbs and pile them into a clean, dry glass jar, before pouring over enough of the vodka to cover them. Leave it to steep until the calendula flowers have opened, then add at least ten of these – you will want to strip the petals from the green bases, chop the whole lot (including the green bases), and pack all of these into the jar with the violets and the vodka. Top up the level of the alcohol if you need to. Leave the resulting combination to infuse for at least another fortnight, longer if possible, then strain out the herbs and bottle the resulting tincture. This can then be diluted by adding 5 ml of the tincture to 10 ml of water. Use as a rinse for the mouth and gums or as a gargle in the case of a sore throat, but do not swallow the remaining liquid.

Violet tea for the bladder

Ingredients
- » 1 part dried violet leaves and flowers (e.g. 10 g)
- » 1 part corn silk (*Zea mays*) (e.g. 10 g)
- » 1 part couch grass (*Agropyron repens*) rhizomes (e.g. 10 g)
- » ½ part dandelion leaf (e.g. 5 g)

Instructions   You will need roughly equal quantities of the dried violet leaves and flowers, corn silk and scrubbed couch grass rhizomes, all finely chopped, and half that quantity of the dandelion leaf – so if you have 10 g each of the first three herbs, allow 5 g of the dandelion leaf. Mix it all up thoroughly and put the herbs into a clean, dry glass jar with an air-tight lid, then label the jar carefully. The dried tea should last at least 6 months – or up to a year, as long as it has a good colour and smells pleasant. Make the tea using 1 tsp, heaped (5 g), of the tea mix to one cup of boiling water and leave it to infuse until it is cool enough to drink. Drink a cup up to three times a day. This can ease bladder infections and make urination a lot more comfortable.

White archangel / white deadnettle
Lamium album

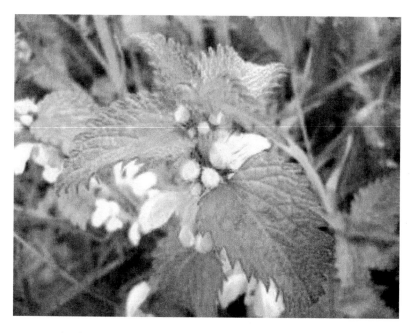

Also known as: blind nettle, dumb nettle, deaf nettle, bee nettle

Family Lamiaceae.

Habitat and description Archangel is quite a low-growing perennial, preferring hedgerows and waysides as well as shady patches in wooded areas. It slightly resembles the stinging nettle; however, it has leaves of a wonderful rich emerald green, roughly spear-shaped, with toothed edges. The leaves somehow look gentler than those of the nettle, less jagged and fierce. The whole plant grows to 20–60 cm (8–24 in). The flowers are a beautiful creamy white, with a vaguely helmeted appearance, like many of the flowers in this particular family, and a velvety look. They form in whorls around a roughly square-shaped hollow stem. The flowers are much loved by bees, and I have to admit I was rather fond of them myself as a child – it is very easy to pluck the flower from its base and suck the nectar from its narrow throat.

Archangel flowers from April through to very late in the autumn – I have even found the odd well-protected plant flowering in December. The whole plant smells quite unpleasant when bruised and is covered with tiny, fine hairs. Many people seem to have a fairly poor opinion of this plant; I, however, consider it much under-rated and under-used. It is actually quite a lovely sight when there are swathes of it in flower, and, of course, it is much loved by bees, as I already mentioned – certainly a good reason to be fond of the plant, given the plight of the bee of late.

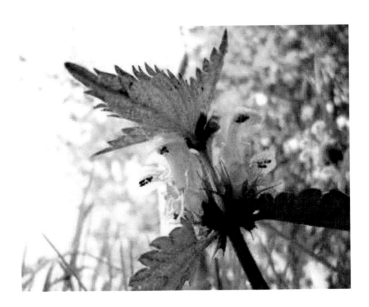

Where to find it   It is commonly found throughout most of Britain except really far north – it isn't quite so fond of the weather in the north of Scotland. It is also found in Ireland and across most of Europe, as well as Asia, as far as Japan, and in North America, where it has naturalised.

Parts used   Leaves and flowers, often separated out for drying.

When to gather   April and May.

Medicines to make   A tea made of the flowers or of the whole young plant tops when just in flower; tincture; infused oil and drawing ointments; poultices; plaisters.

Constituents   Tannins, mucilage; iridoids; phenylpropanoids; flavonol glycosides; flavonoids including quercetin; triterpene saponins; amines such as histamine, choline and tyramine; rosmarinic acid; an alkaloid named lamiine and volatile oils, as well as some potassium salts.

Planetary influence   Venus. (No surprise at all, given its uses!)

Associated deities and heroes   There is very little information on the magical uses of this plant, or on the deities with which it could possibly be associated; however, I'm going to go out on a limb here and hazard a guess that it could be associated with the maiden goddesses – Kore and Persephone, for example. I think any deities linked with an expansive, joyful lightness would be a good fit as well.

Festival   Probably Ostara and Beltane.

Constitution   Warm and dry.

Actions and indications   Culpeper says that white archangel "makes the head merry, drives away melancholy, quickens the spirits, is good against quartan agues, stancheth bleeding at the mouth and nose". Quite a list of recommendations, and it doesn't end there! He also declares that it is good for gout, sciatica and other joint problems, is a good wound healer and is useful in the treatment of ulcers that have gone sour. Finally, he mentions that it can be used to draw out of the skin splinters and other things that should not be stuck there. Gerard comments that the flowers are used to make a distilled water that "makes the heart merry" and "restores the spirits" – an indication of its use in the past as a nervine, perhaps? I can certainly attest that the flowers drunk as a tea are delicious, bringing about a lightness of spirit and even, in some cases, an almost giddy sense of joy, perfect for those prone to being too rooted, heavy and earth-bound, and also for those weighed down by the cares of the world. For this, 1 tsp of the fresh flowers can be brewed up to three times to give increasingly strong infusions.

White archangel is a tonic herb, specifically for the urinary and reproductive tract and the prostate, and, since it is astringent, it is useful for any condition of the respiratory and reproductive tract that generates excessive amounts of catarrh. It is also a mild diuretic, antispasmodic and sedative, as well as a blood cleanser useful in the treatment of spots, acne and pimples.

It is predominantly used as a herb for women's issues, as it is drying and can be used to resolve various problems relating to menstruation. It can be used as a menstrual regulator, to treat excessive and painful bleeding and leucorrhoea. Its histamine, choline and tyramine constituents give this plant its anti-haemorrhagic effect, similar to that of shepherd's purse (*Capsella bursa-pastoris*). As it is astringent, it gives better tone to the uterine tract and is useful for menstrual problems associated with stress, hormone imbalance and related issues.

Archangel has a long-standing reputation as being useful as a venous tonic, to promote tissue healing and act as an anti-inflammatory, possibly due to its flavonoid content.

Some authors are of the opinion that this herb is particularly suited to thin, pale young women whose weakness is brought on by nutritional deficiency.

The fresh young leaves can be steamed with spring onions as a spring vegetable. The flowers make a wonderful tea, picked and infused in hot water, then sweetened with honey, if preferred.

Folklore   The name "*Lamium*" comes from the Greek "*laimos*", meaning "throat", referring to the shape of the flower. The nickname of "archangel" – which I generally use as a matter of course – refers to the plant's general blossoming date of 8 May, a day dedicated to the Archangel Michael.

Dose   Of the tincture, 5 ml three times a day; 2 tsp of the herb per cup of hot water, three times a day.

Contraindications   White archangel is generally safe for all. No contraindications have been found thus far.

White archangel recipes

White archangel spring joy tea

Ingredients
- » plenty of white archangel flowers
- » hot water

Instructions   I recommend gathering these flowers on a sunny day in late April or May – you may even choose to pick the whole flowering plant and separate the flowers from the stems. Try to get them without any green base attached if possible – if you pinch them between thumb and finger, they should come away without any great difficulty. Put the flowers into a shallow basket, and bundle up the leaves and stems with an elastic band before you hang them up to dry. The flowers should dry fairly quickly and are almost as good dry as they are fresh. To make the fresh tea, allow 15 flowers to a mug of hot water, in a cafetiere or teapot. Leave them to infuse until the tea goes a lovely green-gold colour, then pour it into a mug and drink it. This tea doesn't usually need any sweetening, as it is delicious as it is. You can easily enough add a fresh batch of water to the same flowers to make tea to drink through the day, with each batch of flowers giving three rounds of infusion with, oddly enough, increasing strength. If you are using dried flowers, allow 1 tsp of flowers to one mug of water, and drink it in much the same way.

White archangel uplifting elixir

Ingredients
- » plenty of white archangel flowers – at least ¼ pint if possible, the more the better
- » limeflowers
- » rose petals
- » five rosemary leaves
- » vodka
- » honey or maple syrup

Instructions   Add the freshly picked white archangel flowers to a Kilner jar and pour over plenty of vodka and as much honey as you like to give a sweet flavour. Later in the season you can add the limeflowers and the rose petals, and 5 finely chopped rosemary leaves. The idea with the rosemary is to include the uplifting effects without the flavour totally dominating the elixir. Once the final herbs have been added, make sure the alcohol well and truly covers the plant matter and leave the whole thing to infuse for a fortnight before straining the alcohol into a separate bottle. You can put this into a dropper bottle if you want to, and take one dropperful when you are feeling low or overly rooted, to encourage a lightness of spirit. Make sure you label the elixir carefully.

White archangel uterine tonic

Ingredients
- » up to 10 stems of white archangel
- » raspberry leaves: dried leaves, if necessary
- » lemon balm
- » vodka

Instructions   Finely chop the white archangel and pile it into the Kilner jar, along with 20 g of raspberry leaves; dried leaves can be bought online, or you can dry them yourself if you have access to wild raspberry (*Rubus idaeus*). Cover the herbs with enough alcohol to allow an extra 2.5 cm (1 in) on top, and leave it to infuse until the lemon balm is just about to flower. Cut at least 12 stems of lemon balm and finely chop them before adding them to the vodka and herbs – top up the vodka if you need to, to make sure the alcohol covers the herbs. Leave the mixture to infuse for two weeks before straining it. Take 5 ml of the resulting tonic blend up to three times a day as a uterine tonic to help with heavy menstrual bleeding and period pain, as well as easing the symptoms of PMS.

White archangel flower elixir

Ingredients
- » 1 pint of loosely packed white archangel flowers
- » 20 ml maple syrup
- » vodka

Instructions   This one is very easy indeed – just roughly chop the flowers using a mezzaluna and pile them into a Kilner jar; cover with the vodka, before stirring in 20 ml of maple syrup. Leave the whole lot to infuse for at least a fortnight before you strain out the herbs and bottle the elixir. Take 5 ml when you feel your mood starting to slip, before depression really kicks in, or combine it with other treatments and lifestyle changes for the relief of depression. This is a lovely mid-winter tonic when SAD kicks in, as it really reminds you of the joys of spring air and sunshine. Spring will return, even if it doesn't feel like it in midwinter.

Wood avens
Geum urbanum

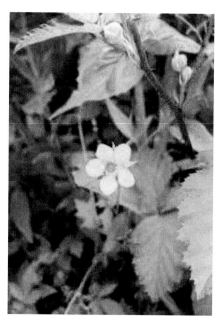

Also known as: herb bennett, colewort, city avens, way bennet,
goldy star of the earth, clove root

Family   Rosaceae.

Habitat and description   Wood avens is commonly found
growing, as the name suggests, in wooded and shady areas; it
doesn't stop there, though, and will often tuck itself into gravel,
flower beds, meadows, under hedges and anywhere else it can
get its feet down. It produces a basal rosette of ruffled green
leaves that don't greatly resemble the leaves on the adult plant,
beginning with pinnate, ruffled leaves in a central whorl, and
leading later on to separate long leaflets that connect to the

main stem. The leaves are lightly hairy and don't smell of much. It has thin, tough stems that grow mostly upright, producing starlike yellow flowers and later on, round, bristly seed heads with hooks on the end of each seed, allowing the seeds to separate from one another and hook onto passers-by. The root is the bit we are particularly interested in, and in wood avens these form clusters of golden yellow, slender tendrils, which have an intriguing clove, ginger and wood-smoke fragrance when unearthed. These tendrils form off a central rhizome, which can be up to 5 cm (2 in.) long. Unlike most root herbs, this plant is unearthed in the spring, particularly after a few dry days in April, which really intensifies the fragrance and flavour.

Where to find it   Europe, the Middle East, and naturalised in North America.

Parts used   Roots predominantly, though the leaves can also be used – they do not have any fragrance, however.

When to gather   March and April: old physicians were adamant that wood avens had to be picked on the 25th of March, on a dry day – though in the damper parts of the world we'll be lucky if the weather is favourable enough then. I've dug for it in April and May to no ill effect – just ensure you dig

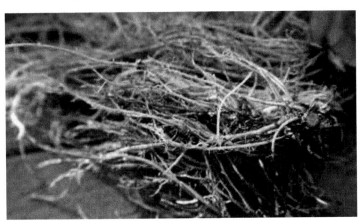

the root before the plant flowers, to get the best levels of fragrance from it.

Medicines to make   Infusions and decoctions, tinctures and elixirs.

Constituents   Tannins and essential oils, plus glycosides.

Planetary influence   Jupiter.

Associated deities and heroes   Any deities linked with triple aspects, such as the Triple Goddess. The Great Mother.

Festival   Midsummer.

Constitution   Warm and dry.

Actions and indications   This is one of those herbs that grows readily in the UK and has been rather overlooked, which is a shame. Wood avens provides a really useful digestive and aromatic, gently bitter tonic for the stomach, particularly for those who run cold and damp, with more "boggy" systems that produce too much mucus and phlegm. I've also used it for diarrhoea due to lax intestinal tone, where it will help to restore balance and encourage more normal bowel movements; it has also been used instead of quinine for intermittent fevers, for which it has quite a reputation. Chew the root to sweeten the breath. The hot infusion of the root is comforting for colds and catarrh, especially for rhinitis after a cold. Create a cold infusion or decoction to use as a gargle for sore throats. A wash made of the infusion or decoction can be used topically for the skin, for spots and freckles – just dab it on with a clean, dry cloth.

Drunk after flu or severe cold, it can dry up excess mucus and relieve a cold, damp stomach, where there is a lot of phlegm causing disordered appetite and nausea, to boost the appetite and improve digestive powers.

The herb and root can also be infused in oil to make a healing balm or a wash for cuts and grazes, very handy for gardener's hands and related issues. I suspect it could also be used in balms for rheumatism and arthritis for its warming properties, and alongside St John's wort for nerve issues where there is inflammation and soreness.

As it is anti-inflammatory and healing, it can also be used for cystitis and other inflammatory conditions around the body. The tannins give it some properties in drying up excessive menstrual bleeding.

The plant is astringent; it is soothing and a warming stomach tonic. It is deobstruant to the liver and spleen, helping to dissolve blockages, and it soothes mucous membranes.

Folklore   This pretty plant has quite a lot of folklore attached to it. The name "herb bennet" is a slurring of "herba benedicta" or "benedict's herb". The botanical name of "geum" (Greek "*geno*", meaning pleasant scented) refers to the fragrance of the roots when they are unearthed. It has been used to ward off evil spirits and venomous creatures and has also been worn as an amulet for the same purposes. Some of the old herbal manuscripts held that it was powerful enough to deter the devil himself. One old legend links it with St Benedict, the saint who was holy enough to drive out poison from a toxic cup merely by holding it. In the medieval era the plant was so beloved and so linked with the church that for a long time it was used as an architectural decoration.

Dose   As a decoction, a cup up to three times a day. Of the cottage tincture, 5 ml up to three times a day.

Contraindications   None known at present.

Wood avens recipes

Preparing and storing wood avens root

Wood avens is one of the few roots we might make use of in the spring, the only other one being dandelion. The root can be a bit of a nuisance to clean and prepare, but the fragrance makes it well worth it. You will need to try to dig the root up on a dry day, ideally once there have been a few warm days, as this concentrates the fragrance. Unearth the root before the plant has flowered, as by this point it has used all of its stored nutrients to fuel the creation of flowers and, later on, seeds. Shake off as much soil as you can, and then give the plant a good wash under an outdoor tap or in a stream, to wash off as much of the excess soil as possible and to remove any little passengers. Then use sharp kitchen scissors to remove the golden root tendrils. This is the part we use most for medicine. Bring them inside and give them another good wash, using a toothbrush to get into any little nooks and crannies. Finely chop the roots, and at this point if you want to dry them, they can go into a very low oven for a long period of time. Alternatively roll them in a tea towel before you chop them, after which you may find they'll dry fairly well laid out on a clean tea towel in a wicker basket. If you dry the roots, you can store them in a clean, dry, air-tight jar, or if you prefer, you can freeze them. Either half fill ice-cube trays with chopped roots, or put teaspoonfuls onto a clean plastic tray, freeze them, then remove them and store them in a labelled jar or pot in the freezer.

Wood avens and sweet cicely digestive tonic

Ingredients
- » ¼ pint of fresh wood avens root
- » ¼ pint of fresh sweet cicely root
- » peppermint leaves, fresh or dried; or tea bags (provided they are good quality)
- » fennel seeds
- » vodka or brandy, depending on preference

Instructions   Finely chop the cleaned, scrubbed roots into small pieces, and do the same with the peppermint, then use a mortar and pestle to crush the fennel seeds and pile all the ingredients into a glass jar before pouring over enough alcohol to cover the herbs, allowing an extra 2.5 cm (1 in.) on top. Leave the whole lot to infuse for at least a fortnight, then strain out the herbs, labelling the resulting liquid carefully. Take 1 tsp (5 ml) up to three times a day to act as a warming digestive tonic, to encourage better digestion of food and an improved appetite. For a depleted appetite, try taking digestive bitters half an hour before meals as well.

Wood avens decoction

Ingredients
» 1 tbsp of finely chopped wood avens root
» 300 ml (10 fl oz) of water

Instructions   Decoctions work beautifully for more woody, fibrous plant parts, in particular roots and suchlike, and in this case boiling up the root makes for a delicious beverage that has elements of spice, smoke and a faint hint of fallen autumn leaves. You will need a stainless steel or enamel saucepan. Place the finely chopped, clean roots and the water into the pan, and bring the mixture up to a boil. Cover with the lid to keep the fragrant steam in, then let it bubble for at least 10 minutes, until the water content has reduced down by a third, then strain out the roots. Drink the resulting decoction in half-cup doses for a cold digestive system with a poor appetite and wind and bloating after meals. This decoction is also a lovely pick-me-up while suffering from the more unpleasant colds and flu.

Wood avens milk infusion

Ingredients
- » 1 tbsp of finely chopped wood avens root
- » 300 ml (10 fl oz) of cow's milk or milk substitute – almond works well

Instructions   As with the decoction, the roots need to be thoroughly cleaned and finely chopped, then simmered gently in the almond milk or milk for at least half an hour. Sweeten the mixture to taste and then enjoy it hot. The digestive benefits of this are similar to those of the decoction, but it will be better suited to those who tend towards cold, dry constitutions, as milk often encourages the production of phlegm. It is, however, a lovely alternative to the traditional golden milk made with the addition of turmeric.

Wood avens balm

Ingredients
- » ½ pint, at least, of loosely packed wood avens leaves
- » 2–3 tbsp of clean, surface-dry wood avens root
- » organic seed oil
- » beeswax pellets
- » clove essential oil
- » bay essential oil

Instructions   Once you have washed the freshly dug wood avens root, use a pair of sharp kitchen scissors or a short, sharp knife to remove the long golden side roots from the main rhizome (discard or compost the woody rhizome itself). Make sure the roots are thoroughly clean, then lay them out in a single layer on a clean, dry tea towel. Carefully roll the tea towel up, trying to keep the roots more or less in a single layer, then roll it vigorously against a kitchen counter or table, much as you would roll a rolling pin over the top of pastry. Unroll the tea towel and check your roots – they should be much more dry after this. Using a mezzaluna, finely chop the wood avens roots and pile them into the top of a double boiler, following them with the finely chopped leaves and enough seed oil to cover the plant matter, allowing an extra 0.5 cm on top of the herbs. Bring the double boiler to a gentle simmer and allow the mixture to heat through for at least half an hour.

If you have a small slow cooker used for infused oil making, this could be a great recipe for that method as well; alternatively, you could use the "sealed tin in a water bath" method where you pile the herbs and oil into a heat-tolerant pot, cover it, and then stand it in a water bath in a low oven, and leave it to heat overnight or all day.

Once the oil has attained that distinctive wood avens fragrance, filter it through either clean muslin or a piece of kitchen roll, then return it to the double boiler, adding 12 g of beeswax per 100 ml (3½ fl oz) of oil. Heat the mixture up, stirring every now and then, until the wax has melted and emulsified with the oil, then add 4 drops each of clove and bay essential oils per 100 ml (3½ fl oz) of oil. Stir it briefly, and pour the mixture into clean, dry glass jars. Once set, label it carefully and store it out of direct sunlight.

This balm is lovely for sore joints and muscles. You can also omit the clove and bay oils and instead use chamomile or lavender to make a balm suitable for cuts and grazes.

Wood avens cottage tincture

Ingredients
- » plenty of finely chopped wood avens roots
- » wood avens leaves
- » brandy

Instructions   You can make this recipe up either as a single tincture or as two separate ones, one made with the leaves and one with the roots. If making a single tincture, with both the roots and the leaves, then scrub and finely chop the wood avens roots — you don't need to worry about drying them in this case, as there will be water content in the alcohol anyway. Pile the finely diced roots into a clean preserving jar and add the finely diced leaves, allowing about twice the amount of leaves to root. Pour over enough brandy to cover the herbs, and put the lid on. This will need to be shaken up every other day for the next fortnight, after which time the herbs can be strained out and the resulting tincture labelled. Take 1 tsp (5 ml) up to three times a day as a digestive tonic or to speed recovery after severe colds or influenza.

Recommended reading

For those wanting to continue their explorations into the ancient healing arts of herbalism, here is a list of books that I thoroughly recommend as being enlightening, inspiring and entertaining to read. This is really just a very brief list – there are so many excellent books out there that I haven't yet stumbled across that I have no doubt the list could easily be three times as long!

Alchemical Medicine for the 21st Century – Spagyrics for Detox, Healing and Longevity
Clare Goodrick-Clarke
ISBN 978-1-59477-913-8
This is a superb, accessible guide to making your own spagyric tinctures, written in language that is comprehensive yet approachable. If you want to have a go at this elaborate and fascinating procedure, this book will give you an excellent jumping-off point.

A Modern Herbal
Mrs M. Grieve
ISBN 1-90477-901-8
This is one of the grandmothers of herb books, and is an immense tome. Worth getting for any herbal historian.

A Woman's Book of Herbs
Elisabeth Brooke
ISBN 978–1–91159–722–3
Beautifully written and inspiring; particularly well suited to those with a more feminist mindset.

Complete Earth Medicine Handbook
Susanne Fischer-Rizzi
ISBN 1–40270–430–5
One of the most beautiful herb books I have ever seen – illustrated with whimsical pencil sketches throughout, and covering some of the more unusual herbs, with some fascinating recipes.

Hedgerow Medicine
Julie Bruton Seal and Matthew Seal
ISBN 978–1–87367–499–4
Covering many of our more common hedgerow herbs and illustrated with a plethora of beautiful photographs.

Herb Craft – A Guide to the Shamanic and Ritual Use of Herbs
Susan Lavender and Anna Franklin
ISBN 1–89830–757–9
If you are interested in the more magical side of plants, this is the book for you.

Practical Herbs 1 / Practical Herbs 2
Henriette Kress
ISBN 978–1–91159–757–5 / 978–1–91159–758–2
Henriette Kress has been an internet staple for many a year now, and was definitely an influence when I was first training. These two books of hers are superb – approachable and full of useful information.

The Earthwise Herbal – A Complete Guide to Old World Medicinal Plants /
The Earthwise Herbal – A Complete Guide to New World Medicinal Plants
Matthew Wood
ISBN 978–1–55643–692–5 / ISBN 978–1–55643–779–3
Matthew Wood needs no real introduction to any herb lover, and his two books are worthy of a place on any herbalist's shelf. Packed full of information, with more specific indications for each plant.

The Herbal Medicine Maker's Handbook – A Home Manual
James Green
ISBN 978–0–89594–990–5
A comprehensive guide to an array of different medicine-making skills, and written in a highly engaging fashion.

The Language of Plants – A Guide to the Doctrine of Signatures
Julia Graves
ISBN 978–1–58420–098–7
For those wanting to gain a more thorough understanding of the Doctrine of Signatures and how to use it as a road map, this is an excellent book.

The Medicinal Flora of Britain and Northwestern Europe
Julian Barker
ISBN 1–87458–163–0
Featuring almost all the wild flowers growing throughout the UK and Europe, this is recommended for anyone wanting to gain information on some of the more weird and wonderful of our medicinal plants.

Weeds in the Heart
Nathanial Hughes and Fiona Owen
ISBN 978–1–91159–748–3
This is a veritable spellbook of herbs, full of the most stunning illustrations and beautifully written.

Witchcraft Medicine – Healing Arts, Shamanic Practices and Forbidden Plants
Claudia Muller Ebeling, Christian Ratsch and Wolf-Dieter Storl
ISBN 978–0–89281–971–3
This book takes your mind places. If you would like to better understand the place of plants for our ancestors, this is a book you may want to delve into.

Index